THE SHARPBRAINS GUIDE TO BRAIN FITNESS

18 Interviews with Scientists, Practical Advice, and Product Reviews, to Keep Your Brain Sharp

NOV 15 2011

Alvaro Fernandez AND Dr. Elkhonon Goldberg

ISBN: 0-9823629-0-0
ISBN-13: 9780982362907
LCCN: 2009900171

Visit www.sharpbrains.com to order additional copies.

We dedicate this book to your Unique Brain, and your Unique Mind.

Table of Contents

Foreword

In the winter of 2007, as I was planning a new conference titled "Brain Health Across The Lifespan" with the Institute on Aging, I recognized the growing interest in the topic of brain fitness. This felt like a breath of fresh air.

During my 30 years leading the American Society on Aging we focused heavily on the importance of lifelong learning and mental stimulation as an important component of healthy aging. Now that scientists know more about the lifelong neuroplasticity of our brains, and how our lifestyles, actions and thoughts influence the way our brains develop with age, newspapers, magazines, TV, and books, are enthusiastically covering the field of brain fitness and "brain training".

Widespread media coverage, though, combined with often contradictory or partial product claims, has contributed to confusion in the minds of some consumers and professionals as to how to navigate the growing array of options. Is doing one more crossword puzzle the best thing I can do for my brain? Or is it taking some vitamin supplements? Why are both physical and mental exercises so important, and complementary to each other? Why is managing stress as critical to cognitive health as, say, finding stimulating activities to do? What is the value of new "brain training games," and how can I evaluate and compare them?

For the Brain health Across The Lifespan conference, I wanted to bring the best speaker and resources on the topic of brain fitness. Asking around dozens of colleagues, I came to hear the name SharpBrains over and over – peers mentioned how Dr. Elkhonon Goldberg and Alvaro Fernandez, co-founders of SharpBrains and co-authors of this guide, had been providing much-needed quality information about the growing field of brain fitness. This is why I invited Alvaro Fernandez to speak at our conference in 2008 and why I am honored to write this foreword.

Neuroscientist Dr. Elkhonon Goldberg and educator and executive Alvaro Fernandez have been working for years with dozens of scientists and experts to answer questions like those above. They founded SharpBrains, a market research company that covers the healthcare and educational applications of neuroscience, to provide information and services to its impressive roster of clients, including leading healthcare providers, insurance companies, universities, and more. I am pleased that they have now distilled much information and advice into this practical and thought-provoking guide.

I am sure that you will feel more enlightened, stimulated, and hopeful, after reading the eye-opening book you have in your hands - as I do.

Gloria Cavanaugh, former President and CEO of the American Society on Aging and founding Board member of the National Alliance for Caregiving.

Introduction:

Debunking 10 Brain and Brain Fitness Myths

You are a lifelong learner. You may also be a caregiver, or a professional in fields such as healthcare, education, or psychology. The goal of this guide is to help you make informed decisions about brain health and cognitive fitness, based on latest scientific findings. With this guide, the first of its kind, we want to help you navigate the growing number of studies, new products and confusing myths and claims that are part of the emerging brain fitness field.

Only two years ago, the word "brain" would have rarely been seen next to "fitness" or "training". Today, not a week goes by without a significant media report or announcement linking those precise words.

The flood of recent global news coverage on brain fitness and brain training reflects a growing interest in natural, non drug-based interventions to keep our brains sharp as we age. This interest is very timely, given an aging population, increasing life span, increasing prevalence of Alzheimer's rates, a complex changing environment that places more lifelong cognitive demands on our brains than ever and soaring health care costs in the U.S. that place emphasis on prevention and lifestyle changes.

2007 was a turning point for the brain fitness field with a jump in media coverage throughout the year. The first notable press coverage was a Time/CNN special in January 2007. In June, a full issue of the *Journal of Gerontology* was devoted to cognitive training. The year ended with a PBS special titled

"The Brain Fitness Program" in December. Why is this happening? There were significant scientific breakthroughs linking cognitive training to lasting cognitive improvements. Multiple studies were published (including the ACTIVE and IMPACT studies examined in depth later in this guide) that showed a clear causal relationship between cognitive training and cognitive improvements. Products like Nintendo's Brain Age sold millions of copies worldwide. Popular books on the topic, like *Wall Street Journal* columnist Sharon Begley's *Train Your Mind, Change Your Brain, and The Brain That Changes Itself* by Norman Doidge made it to the *New York Times'* Best Seller list.

Not only that. Throughout the year, brain fitness software providers got endorsements from and made partnerships with government entities, healthcare providers and insurance companies. For example, neuroscientist Dr. Susan Greenfield, Director of the Royal Institution in England, endorsed a commercially available product MindFit. Humana, a leading health insurance company, rolled out an agreement to offer Posit Science's brain fitness program to Humana Medicare members.

At the same time, the rapid growth of this emerging field is resulting in major confusion among consumers and professionals alike.

For instance, in November and December of 2008, two scientific studies have questioned widespread assumptions: one of them showed how popular plant supplement *Ginkgo biloba* does not prevent cognitive decline or halt progress to Alzheimer's disease. The other one, in contrast, showed how playing complex videogames may significantly help older brains.

The evidence supporting the direct efficacy of many of the available brain training products is yet lacking. As Dr. Kramer, an expert in brain fitness and physical exercise, points out "It is true that some companies are being more science-based than others; but, in my view, the consumer-oriented field is growing faster than the research is." Dr. Jensen, who has written twenty-one books on the brain and learning, adds "I see too many books saying 'brain' in the title that are not grounded in any brain research. Something I always recommend when shopping for books is to check the references section, making sure the book references specific studies in credible journals since 2000."

Moreover, we need better definitions, a better taxonomy of key concepts. As we emphasize in this guide, mental exercise or "brain training" goes beyond mental activity. It refers to the structured use of cognitive exercises or techniques aimed at improving specific brain functions. Yet, this level of analysis is often missing in popular media coverage.

There are many current and potential applications of brain training beyond healthy aging. For starters, what about safer driving among teenagers and older adults? Further, there are a variety of clinical conditions (including strokes and traumatic brain injury) for which non-invasive, computerized cognitive training programs can play a role both as first line interventions and post diagnosis to complement existing treatments.

This first guide is the result of over a year of extensive research including interviews with more than a hundred scientists, professionals and consumers. We hope it proves to be a worthy resource.

The SharpBrains Guide to Brain Fitness is organized into seven chapters. Chapter 1 takes you inside a brain and show you how neuroplasticity is at the core of brain fitness. Chapter 2 describes the four pillar of brain maintenance: balanced nutrition, stress management, physical exercise and mental stimulation. Chapter 3 delves deeper into mental exercise, and shows the different ways in which mental exercise can deliver results that go beyond the benefits of daily mental activity. Chapter 4 offers tools to navigate through the brain training software programs available, and includes our 21 Quick Picks. Chapter 5 reviews a range of current and future applications of brain training. Chapter 6 synthesizes a number of emerging trends, so you are better prepared for the future. Finally, Chapter 7 opens the current debate to you, your friends, loved ones, colleagues, neighbors.

In this guide you will also find transcripts of interviews with prominent scientists that provide in depth reviews of the scientific topics covered. These interviews were conducted by Alvaro Fernandez, Co-Founder and CEO of SharpBrains, from September 2006 until November 2008.

Finally, please note that we do not prescribe or endorse any specific brain training programs. This guide aspires to offer research-based, relevant and up-to-date information and tools. We leave it to you to exercise your brain and make appropriate decisions.

DEBUNKING 10 BRAIN AND BRAIN FITNESS MYTHS

MYTHS	FACTS
1. Genes determine the fate of our brains.	Lifelong neuroplasticity allows our lifestyles and actions to play a meaningful role in how our brains physically evolve, especially given longer life expectancy.
2. Aging means automatic decline.	There is nothing inherently fixed in the precise trajectory of how brain functions evolve as we age.
3. Medication is the main hope for cognitive enhancement.	Non-invasive interventions can have comparable and more durable effects, side effect-free.
4. We will soon have a Magic Pill or General Solution to solve all our cognitive challenges.	A multi-pronged approach is recommended, centered around nutrition, stress management, and both physical and mental exercise.
5. There is only one "it" in "Use It or Lose it".	The brain is composed of a number of specialized units. Our life and productivity depend on a variety of brain functions, not just one.
6. All brain activities or exercises are equal.	Varied and targeted exercises are the necessary ingredients in brain training so that a wide range of brain functions can be stimulated.
7. There is only one way to train your brain.	Brain functions can be impacted in a number of ways: through meditation, cognitive therapy, cognitive training.
8. We all have something called "Brain Age".	Brain age is a fiction. No two individuals have the same brain or expression of brain functions.
9. That "brain age" can be reversed by 10, 20, 30 years.	Brain training can improve specific brain functions, but, with research available today, cannot be said to roll back one's "brain age" by a number of years.
10. All human brains need the same brain training.	As in physical fitness, users must ask themselves: What functions do I need to improve on? In what timeframe? What is my budget?

We would like to thank Dr. Pascale Michelon, Research Manager for this guide, and the dozens of people who have shared their time and perspectives with us.

Alvaro Fernandez,
Co-Founder & CEO, SharpBrains
Dr. Elkhonon Goldberg,
Co-Founder and Chief Scientific Advisor, SharpBrains

Chapter 1.
The Brain and Brain Fitness 101

HIGHLIGHTS

- The brain is composed of a number of specialized regions serving distinct functions.
- Our life and productivity depend on a variety of brain functions, not just one.
- There is nothing inherently fixed in the trajectory of how brain functions evolve as we age.

In order to make informed decisions about brain health and brain training, you need to first understand the underlying organization of the human brain and how it evolves across our lifespan.

1.1. BRAIN STRUCTURES

The dominant structure of the human brain is called the cerebrum, which consists of the grey, curly cortex. The cerebrum is divided into two hemispheres (right and left), each consisting of four lobes, and controls higher mental functions. As you can see in Figure 1, the four lobes of the brain are the occipital, temporal, parietal and frontal lobes.

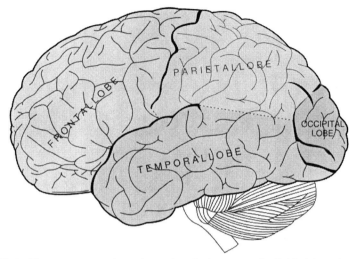

FIGURE 1: The cortex consists of two hemispheres, each divided into four lobes: frontal, parietal, occipital and temporal.

The cortex includes a number of neurons or brain cells (see Figure 2). These neurons communicate through connection, called synapses. An average brain contains approximately 100 billions neurons. But other types of cells, called glial cells, also play an important role.

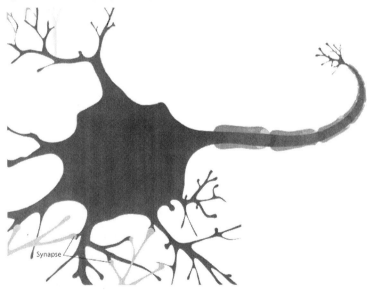

FIGURE 2: This is a neuron. Your brain contains approximately 100 billions of these. Neurons communicate through synapses.

Different areas of the brain are responsible for different functions.

The frontal lobes (behind the forehead) are primarily responsible for decision-making, planning, problem-solving, and certain forms of attention. They are also involved in motor control, certain aspects of language and memory, social behavior and emotions.

The occipital lobes (at the back of the brain) are devoted to vision.

The temporal lobes (next to the temples) are responsible mostly for memory formation, language, hearing and object perception.

The parietal lobes are responsible mostly for certain forms of attention, spatial processing and the manipulation of objects.

1.2. BRAIN FUNCTIONS

You have probably heard about cognitive function or cognition. What is cognition? Cognition has to do with how a person understands and acts in the world. It is a set of processes that are part of nearly every human action. Cognitive abilities are the brain-based skills we need to carry out any task – from the simplest to the most complex. They have more to do with the mechanisms of how we learn, remember, problem-solve, and pay attention rather than with any actual knowledge. Any task can be broken down into the different cognitive skills or functions needed to complete that task successfully.

The fields of neuropsychology, cognitive psychology, and thus cognitive training are based on the framework that cognition consists of different mental functions which are based on specific constellations of brain structures. In Table 1, you can browse through the main brain functions involved in cognition. For more discussion on one specific brain function, attention, see the interview at the end of this chapter with Dr. Posner, a pioneer in this area.

BRAIN FUNCTION	SKILLS INVOLVED
Perception	Recognition and interpretation of sensory stimuli.
Attention	Ability to sustain concentration on a particular object, action, or thought. Ability to manage competing demands in our environment.
Memory	Short-term memory (limited storage). Long-term memory (unlimited storage).
Motor	Ability to mobilize our muscles and bodies. Ability to manipulate objects.
Language and Auditory Processing	Skills allowing us to differentiate and comprehend sounds and generate verbal output.
Visual and Spatial Processing	Ability to process incoming visual stimuli. Ability to visualize images and scenarios.
Executive Functions	Abilities that enable goal-oriented behavior, such as the ability to plan, and execute a goal. These include: • Flexibility: the capacity for quickly switching to the appropriate mental mode. • Theory of mind: insight into other people's inner world, their plans, their likes and dislikes. • Anticipation: prediction based on pattern recognition. • Problem-solving: defining the problem in the right way to then generate solutions and pick the right one. • Decision making: the ability to make decisions based on problem-solving, on incomplete information and on emotions (ours and others'). • Working Memory: the capacity to hold and manipulate information "on-line" in real time. • Emotional self-regulation: the ability to identify and manage one's own emotions for good performance. • Sequencing: the ability to break down complex actions into manageable units and prioritize them in the right order. • Inhibition: the ability to withstand distraction, and internal urges.

TABLE 1. The main brain functions involved in cognition.

1.3. THE AGING BRAIN

As we age, our whole body changes. The same is true for the brain. The most common structural change is brain atrophy as neurons, and mostly connections between neurons, die. In terms of functional changes, age-related cognitive decline typically starts at about forty when the brain processing speed slows down.

Dr. Jerri Edwards, whose interview you will find at the end of Chapter 5, defines processing speed as "mental quickness". Younger brains process information faster than older brains. Young and old brains can accomplish the same tasks but the older brains will do so more slowly. In our daily life, the speed at which we process incoming information can be crucial. This is the case for instance when one is driving and has to assess the situation and take decision in a 1/45th of a second.

Along with speed of processing, other brain functions decline over time. The decline typically happens in areas that underlie our capacity to learn and adapt to new environments, such as problem-solving in novel situations, memory, attention, mental imagery, vision, hearing, dexterity and flexibility. Generally, getting older reduces both one's ability to focus and the capacity for learning new information. As we age, it takes more and more inhibition skills to tune out distractions and stay focused. Of course, individuals vary in how and when they experience these decreases, but they will eventually occur.

At the same time, growing older generally means that one has acquired more knowledge and wisdom. Indeed, some functions do tend to improve with age, such as vocabulary and other word-related language skills, pattern recognition and emotional self-regulation. In general, skills that depend heavily on accumulated experience tend to improve. Wisdom can be seen as the ability that enables us to solve problems efficiently, develop empathy and insight, and refine moral reasoning. For example, as judges tackle more complex cases, they develop wisdom or an intuition for solutions and strategies.

In sum, as long as the environment does not change too rapidly, we tend to continue to accumulate valid wisdom throughout our lives, yet our capacity to process and deal with change declines.

1.4. NEUROPLASTICITY

In the past decade there has been a fundamental change in our understanding of human brain capacity. New research from scientists at the Salk Institute, the Karolinska Institute, Columbia University and elsewhere has given a renewed, positive view of the human brain and its potential for change and development throughout life.

The human brain is now considered to be a highly dynamic and constantly reorganizing system capable of being shaped and reshaped across an entire lifespan. It is believed that every experience alters the brain's organization at some level. The key words in this new approach to the brain are neuroplasticity and neurogenesis. Neuroplasticity refers to the lifelong capacity of the brain to change and rewire itself in response to the stimulation of learning and experience. Neurogenesis is the ability to create new neurons and connections between neurons throughout a lifetime. The latter process is also referred to as synaptogenesis. Neuroscientists often tend to distinguish between "neurogenesis" and "synaptogenesis", but for reasons of simplicity we will refer to both with a combined term "neurogenesis." This new paradigm contrasts with traditional ideas of the human brain being a fixed and essentially limited system that only degrades with age.

As we age, the rate of change in the brain, or neuroplasticity, declines but does not come to a halt. In addition, we now know that new neurons can appear in certain parts of the brain up until the day we die.

Brain plasticity is the ability that brain training takes advantages of to try to slow down the aging process. Brain plasticity is also crucial following head injury. It is the one brain's ability that allows recovery. For an example of a spectacular recovery see the interview, at the end of this chapter, with Lee Woodruff whose husband suffered a severe traumatic brain injury in Iraq.

Recently, brain changes as a result of cognitive activity have been observed directly in the brain thanks to brain imaging. Brain imaging allows scientists to produce images of the brain that show its structure, as well as where in the brain activity is taking place as it is engaged in various cognitive activities. New neuroimaging methods have changed neuroscience in the same way that the telescope changed astronomy. There are different types of brain imaging:

structural and functional. Structural imaging provides information about the shape and volume of the brain through computed axial tomography (CAT) and magnetic resonance imaging (MRI) scans. Functional imaging, such as functional magnetic resonance imaging (fMRI) and positron emission tomography (PET) scans, shows the brain regions that are active when one performs a specific task.

Evidence of neuroplasticity has been observed mostly in the brains of individuals who became experts in a particular skill. Why? Because changes associated with learning occur massively when we become expert in a specific domain. The areas of the brain that support the skills at which one has become an expert change over time.

An intriguing study showed that London taxi drivers have a larger hippocampus (in the temporal lobe) than London bus drivers (Maguire, Woollett, & Spiers, 2006). This is explained by the fact that the hippocampus is important for forming and accessing complex memories, including spatial memories necessary to navigate efficiently. Taxi drivers have to navigate around London whereas bus drivers follow a limited set of routes. Thus the hippocampus of taxi driver is particularly stimulated and gets to change over time.

Plasticity can also be observed in the brains of bilinguals (Mechelli et al., 2004). It looks like learning a second language is associated with structural changes in the brain: the left inferior parietal cortex is larger in bilingual brains than in monolingual brains.

Plastic changes also occur in musicians brains compared to non-musicians. Gaser and Schlaug (2003) compared professional musicians (who practice at least 1h per day) to amateur musicians and non-musicians. They found that in several brain areas involved in playing music (motor regions, anterior superior parietal areas and inferior temporal areas) the volume of cortex was highest in professional musicians, intermediate in amateur musicians, and lowest in non-musicians!

A recent study showed that one doesn't need to become an expert to exhibit signs of neuroplasticity. In 2006, Draganski and his colleagues imaged the brains of German medical students 3 months before their medical exam and right after the exam. They compared the brains of these students to the brains of students who were not studying for exam at this time. Medical students' brains showed changes in regions of the parietal cortex as well as in the posterior hippocampus. As you can guess, these regions of the brains are known to be involved in memory and learning. This shows one more time that changes in the brain occur following the experience of learning.

1.5. LIFELONG LEARNING

Learning is the physical process of changing our brains. Today we know this is possible at all ages, bringing the concept and practice of lifelong learning to the forefront.

Learning is thought to be "neuro-protective." Through neuroplasticity, learning increases connections between neurons, increases cellular metabolism, and increases the production of nerve growth factor, a substance produced by the body to help maintain and repair neurons.

When we learn, we create physical changes inside our brains. By practicing a skill, we repeatedly stimulate the same area of the brain, which strengthens existing neural connections and creates new ones (think about the London taxi drivers). Over time, we can become more cognitively efficient, using fewer neurons to do the same job. And the more often we fire up certain mental circuits, the easier it is to get them going again.

Thus learning is critical at all ages to maintain good brain functions. According to neurobiologist Dr. James Zull, whose interview can be found at the end of the present Chapter, one way to motivate ourselves to keep learning is to search for meaningful bridges between what we want to learn and what we already know. When we do so, we cultivate our neuronal networks. "We become our own gardeners."

1.6. WHAT IS BRAIN FITNESS?

Brain fitness is our brain's ability to readily create additional connections between neurons, and even to promote new neurons in certain parts of the brain. Research in neuropsychology and neuroscience shows that vigorous mental activity can lead to good brain fitness, which in turn, translates into a sharper memory, faster processing of information, better attention, and other improved cognitive skills.

In general, brain fitness products are geared to change the trajectory of the life curve so that younger minds improve their peaks (or reach them faster) and older people do not experience such a loss in various cognitive abilities, like mental flexibility, working memory, and others.

If the brain is flexible and molded through experience, the question is, "What tools can help provide the right kind of experience to help refine our brains, from a structural and functional point of view?" The goal of this guide is precisely to help you answer that question.

1.7. INTERVIEWS

- Dr. Michael Posner - What is attention and how to train it.
- Dr. James Zull – What is learning?
- Dr. Eric Jensen – Learning and the brain.
- Dr. Robert Sylwester – Brain development.
- Lee Woodruff – Recovering from traumatic brain injury.

Interview with Dr. Michael I. Posner – What is attention and how to train it.

BACKGROUND:

Michael I. Posner is a prominent scientist in the field of cognitive neuroscience. He is currently an Emeritus Professor of Neuroscience at the University of Oregon (Department of Psychology, Institute of Cognitive and Decision Sciences). In August 2008, the International Union of Psychological Science made him the first recipient of the Dogan Prize in recognition of a contribution that represents a major advance in psychology.

HIGHLIGHTS:

- There is not one single "attention", but three separate functions of attention: alerting, orienting, and executive attention.
- A 5-day intervention aimed at training executive attention in children between 4 and 7 years of age showed that executive attention was trainable.

Dr. Posner, many thanks for your time today. I really enjoyed the James Arthur Lecture monograph on Evolution and Development of Self-Regulation that you delivered last year. Could you provide a summary of the research you presented?

I would emphasize that we human beings can regulate our thoughts, emotions, and actions to a greater degree than other primates. For example, we can choose to pass up an immediate reward for a larger, delayed reward. We can plan ahead, resist distractions, be goal-oriented. These human characteristics appear to depend upon what we often call "self-regulation." What is exciting these days is that progress in neuroimaging and in genetics makes it possible to think about self-regulation in terms of specific brain-based networks.

Can you explain what self-regulation is?

All parents have seen this in their kids. Parents can see the remarkable transformation as their children develop the ability to regulate emotions and to persist with goals in the face of distractions. That ability is usually labeled "self-regulation."

The other main area of your research is attention. Can you explain the brain basis for what we usually call "attention"?

I have been interested in how the attention system develops in infancy and early childhood. One of our major findings, thanks to neuroimaging, is that there is not one single "attention", but three separate functions of attention with three separate underlying brain networks: alerting, orienting, and executive attention.
   1) Alerting: helps us maintain an alert state.
   2) Orienting: focuses our senses on the information we want. For example, you are now listening to my voice.
   3) Executive Attention: regulates a variety of networks, such as emotional responses and sensory information. This is critical for most other skills, and clearly correlated with academic performance. It is distributed in frontal lobes and the cingulate gyrus.

The development of executive attention can be easily observed both by questionnaire and cognitive tasks after about age 3–4, when parents can identify the ability of their children to regulate their emotions and control their behavior in accord with social demands.

"Executive attention" sounds similar to executive functions.

Executive functions are goal-oriented. Executive attention is just the ability to manage attention towards those goals, towards planning. Both are clearly correlated. Executive attention is important for decision-making (how to accomplish an external goal) and with working memory (the temporary storage of information). For example, given that you said earlier that you liked my monograph, I have been thinking of the subheadings and sections there as I provide you my answers, using my working memory capacity.

You said that the three functions of attention are supported by separate neural networks.

Neuroimaging allows us to identify sets of distributed areas that operate together. Different techniques allow us to see different things. For example, fMRI lets us see the activation of areas of grey matter. A more recent technique, diffusion tensor, is focused instead on the white matter. It detects connectivity among neurons, it helps us see a map of networks.

How many networks have been identified so far?

So far, a number of networks have been identified. For an illustration, you can see the wonderful interactive Brain Map by the University of Texas, San Antonio. Let me add another fascinating area of research. There is a type of neuron, named the Von Economo neuron, which is found only in the anterior cingulate and a related area of the anterior insula, very common in humans, less in other primates, and completely absent in most non-primates. These neurons have long axons, connecting to the anterior cingulate and anterior insula, which we think is part of the reason why we have Executive Attention. Diffusion tensor allows us to identify this white matter, these connections across separate brain structures, in the live brain. From a practical point of view, we can think that neural networks like this are what enable specific human traits such as effortful control.

What is effortful control?

It is a higher-order temperament factor consisting of attention, focus shifting, and inhibitory control - both for children and adults. A common example is how often you may make plans that you do not follow through with. A test often used to measure executive attention is the Stroop Test.

Effortful control has been shown to correlate with the scores on executive attention at several ages during childhood, and imaging studies have linked it to brain areas involved in self-regulation. Good parenting has been shown to build good effortful control, so there are clear implications from this research.

Tell us now about your recent research on attention training

Several training programs have been successful in improving attention in normal adults and in patients suffering from different pathologies. With normal adults, training with video games produced better performance on a range of visual attention tasks. Training has also led to specific improvements in executive attention in patients with specific brain injury. Working-memory training can improve attention with ADHD children.

In one recent study we developed and tested a 5-day training intervention using computerized exercises. We tested the effect of training during the period of major development of executive attention, which takes place between 4 and 7 years of age.We found that executive attention was trainable, and also a significantly greater improvement in intelligence in the trained group compared to the control children. This finding suggested that training effects had generalized to a measure of cognitive processing that is far removed from the training exercises.

A collaborator of our lab, Dr. Yiyuan Tang, studied the impact of mindfulness meditation with undergraduates to improve executive attention, finding significant improvements as well. We hope that training methods like this will be further evaluated, along with other methods, both as possible means of improving attention prior to school and for children and adults with specific needs.

Can you explain the potential implications of this emerging research on Education and Health?

It is clear that executive attention and effortful control are critical for success in school. Will they one day be trained in pre-schools? It sounds reasonable to believe so, to make sure all kids are ready to learn. Of course, additional studies are needed to determine exactly how and when attention training can best be accomplished and its lasting importance.

In terms of health, many deficits and clinical problems have a component of serious deficits in executive attention network. For example, when we talk about attention deficits, we can expect that in the future there will be remediation methods, such as working memory training, to help alleviate those deficits.

Let me add that we have found no ceiling for abilities such as attention, including among adults. The more training, even with normal people, the higher the results.

Let me ask your take on that eternal question, the roles of nature and nurture.

There is a growing number of studies that show the importance of interaction between our genes and each of our environments. Epigenetics is going to help us understand that question better, but let me share a very interesting piece of research from my lab where we found an unusual interaction between genetics and parenting.

Good parenting, as measured by different research-based scales, has been shown to build good effortful control which, as we saw earlier, is so important. Now, what we found is that some specific genes reduced, even eliminated, the influence of the quality of parenting. In other words, some children's development really depends on how their parents bring them up, whereas others do not - or do to a much smaller extent.

Too bad that we do not have time now to explore all the potential ethical implications from emerging research like that...let me ask a few final questions. First, given that we have been talking both about formal training programs (computer-based, meditation) and also informal ones (parenting), do we know how formal and informal learning interact? What type can be most effective when, and for whom?

Great question. We don't know at this point. A research institute in Seattle, funded by the National Science Foundation, is trying to address that question. One practical issue they address is the influence of bilingual education on cognition.

How can SharpBrains readers access the computer-based attention training program you talked about earlier?

Researchers and parents can download the program, which is aimed at kids aged 4 to 6. The computerized exercises are available on www.teach-the-brain.org. Click on learning tools and follow attention.

Finally, what can we expect from your lab in the next years?

We will hear soon if we obtain the NIH proposal to train children at age 5 and then follow-up over the years, compared to a control group. The program I mentioned earlier showed good short-term results, but we would like to track those kids over time and see what happens. For example, we will examine whether or not an early intervention might translate into a "snowball effect" of higher levels of cognitive and school performance.

Interview with Dr. James Zull – What is learning?

BACKGROUND:

Dr. James Zull is a Professor of biology and biochemistry at Case Western University. Dr. Zull is also the Director of the University Center for Innovation in Teaching and Education (UCITE) at Case Western.

Dr. Zull loves to learn, teach, and build connections. He has spent years building bridges between neurobiology and pedagogy. His book, *The Art of Changing the Brain: Enriching the Practice of Teaching by Exploring the Biology of Learning,* shows how neurobiological research can inform and refine some of the best ideas in educational theory. In the book, Dr. Zull adds a biological perspective to David Kolb's Learning Cycle framework from his book, *Experiential Learning: Experience as the Source of Learning and Development.* Whereas Kolb reviews human learning, Dr. Zull is focused on how apes go through the same stages when they learn a new activity, activating exactly the same brain areas that we do.

HIGHLIGHTS:

- Every brain can change, at any age, so learning is critical at all ages, not only in the school environment.
- Children need to flex their "learning muscle" – to learn how to learn.
- Schools should focus more on how all kids could learn more.

THE VIRTUOUS LEARNING CYCLE

What is learning? Can apes really learn the same way that humans do?

Learning is physical. Learning means the modification, growth, and pruning of our neuronal networks, through experience. And, yes, we have seen that apes go through the same Learning Cycle that we do, activating the same or similar brain areas.

How does learning happen?

There are 4 stages in the "Learning Cycle:"

Stage One: We have a concrete experience.
Stage Two: We develop reflective observations and connections.
Stage Three: We generate abstract hypotheses
Stage Four: Then we actively test those hypotheses.

In the forth stage, we have a new concrete experience, and a new Learning Cycle ensues. In other words, we get information (activating the sensory cortex), make meaning of that information (in the back integrative cortex), create new ideas from these meanings (in the front integrative cortex), and act on those ideas (using the motor cortex). From this, I propose that there are four pillars of learning: gathering, analyzing, creating, and acting. This is how we learn.

Learning in this way requires effort and getting out of our comfort zones. A key condition for learning is self-driven motivation, a sense of ownership. To feel in control, to feel that one is making progress, is necessary for this Learning

Cycle to self-perpetuate. Antonio Damasio made a strong point about the role of emotions in his engaging book *Descartes' Error.*

HOW TO IMPROVE LEARNING ABILITIES

Can we, as learners, motivate ourselves? How can we become better learners?

Great question, because in fact that is a uniquely human ability. We know that the brain's frontal lobes, which are proportionally much larger in humans than in any other mammals, are key for emotional self-regulation. We can be proactive and identify the areas that motivate us, and build on those. In other words, the "art of the learner" may be the art of finding connections between the new information or challenges and what we already know and care about.

If I had to select one mental muscle that students should really exercise and grow during their school years, I would say they need to build their "learning muscle" – to learn how to learn. That might be even more valuable than learning what we stress in the curriculum, i.e., rote memory and the specific subjects we teach.

Do you think this is happening today in schools?

I do not think so. First, of all, too many people still believe that education means the process by which students passively absorb information. Even if many educators would like to ensure a more participatory and active approach, we still use the structures and priorities of another era. For example, we still pay too much attention to categorizing some kids as intelligent and some as not so intelligent, instead of focusing on how all kids could learn more.

Second, learning and changing are not that easy. Both require effort, and also, by definition, getting out of our comfort zones. We need to try new things, and to fail. The active testing phase is a critical one. Sometimes our hypothesis will be right, and sometimes it will be wrong. The fear of failing, the fear of looking not smart, is a key obstacle to learning that I see too often, especially with people who want to protect perceived reputations to such an extent that they do not let themselves try new learning cycles.

Given what you just said, how do you help your students become better learners?

Despite the fact that every brain is different, let me simplify and say that I usually observe two types of students each with different obstacles to learning and benefiting from different strategies.

1) Introverted Students: Students who have a tendency toward introversion can be very good at the reflection and abstract hypothesis phases, but not so good at the active testing one. In order to change that, I help create small groups where they feel safe and can take risks such as sharing their thoughts aloud and asking questions.

2) Extroverted Students: More extroverted students can be very good at having constant concrete experiences and active testing, but may benefit from increased reflection and abstract hypothesis development. Having them do things like writing papers and predicting the outcome of certain experiments or even current political affairs, helps.

What other tips would you offer to teachers and parents to help children learn?

Always try to provoke an active reaction. This will ensure that the student is engaged and sees the connection between the new information and what he or she already knows. You can do this by asking questions such as "What does this make you think of? Is there some part of this new material that rings a bell for you?"

To ensure a safe learning environment, you have to make sure to accept all answers, and build on them. We should view students as plants and flowers that need careful cultivation: grow some areas, help reduce others.

Please give us an example.

An example I use in my books is that middle school students often have a hard time learning about Martin Luther and the Reformation because they confuse him with Martin Luther King Jr. We can choose to become frustrated about that. Or we can exploit this saying something like, "Yes! Martin Luther King was a lot like Martin Luther. In fact, why do you think Martin Luther King's parents named him that? Why do you think they did not name him Sam King?"

LEARNING AND THE ADULT BRAIN

What would you suggest for adults who want to become better learners?

Learning is critical at all ages, not only in the school environment. We have brains precisely in order to be able to learn, to adapt to new environments. This is essential throughout life, not just when we are in school.

We now know that every brain can change, at any age. There is really no upper limit on learning since the neurons seem to be capable of growing new connections whenever they are used repeatedly. I think all of us need to develop the capacity to motivate ourselves. One way to do that is to search for meaningful contact points and bridges, between what we want to learn and what we already know. When we do so, we cultivate our neuronal networks. We become our own gardeners.

Interview with Eric Jensen – Learning and the brain.

BACKGROUND:

Eric Jensen is a former middle school teacher and former adjunct professor at several universities including the University of California at San Diego. He co-founded the Learning Brain Expo, a conference for educators, and has written twenty-one books on the brain and learning. Jensen is currently completing his PhD coursework. His most recent book, *Enriching the Brain: How to Maximize Every Learner's Potential* (2006), is highly recommended for educators and parents alike. He wrote an article featured in *Phi Delta Kappan* in February 2008 that sparked a healthy debate on the value of neuroscience applied to education.

HIGHLIGHTS:

- There are clear implications from brain research that educators should be aware of. For instance nutrition, physical exercise, stress management, and overall mental enrichment should be focused on instead of being neglected.
- An increasing number of researchers are working with educators to find the best ways to bridge theory and practice.

Can you explain the role that you and your organization play?

We act as translators between the neuroscience and education fields, helping to build a Brain-Based Education movement. We launched the first conference that attempted to bridge these two worlds in 1998. The goal of the conference, called Learning Expo, was for teachers to speak to scientists, and, equally important, for scientists to speak to educators.

Critics say that neuroscience research can add little to educational practices. What we say is that it is true that much needs to be clarified, but there are already clear implications from brain research that educators should be aware of. For example, four important elements that are often neglected by educators, given the obsessive focus on academic scores, are nutrition, physical exercise, stress management, and overall mental enrichment.

Since 1998? How would you characterize the progress so far?

The good news is that today more educators than ever are learning about how the brain works. There are a growing number of academic programs such as Harvard's masters program in Mind, Brain, and Education, and peer-reviewed journals such as the *Mind, Brain and Education* Journal.

Still, there are clear areas for improvement. Too many staff developers are weak on the science. I see too many books saying "brain" in the title that are not grounded in any brain research. Something I always recommend when shopping for books is to check the references section, making sure the book references specific studies in credible journals since 2000.

Now, those are mostly awareness-related initiatives. What, if any, are the implications for daily teaching and learning in schools?

You are right, this is still an emerging field. A number of private, independent, forward-thinking public schools and charter schools are implementing specific initiatives, mostly around brain-based teaching strategies, nutrition and exercise. But these are tougher to implement for some public schools, which have limited resources and flexibility. We also see a growing number of enlightened parents learning about the principles we discuss and applying them at home.

Have you seen any impact at the policy level? Specifically, what do you think about the current debate about the merits or lack thereof of No Child Left Behind?

I agree with the move towards accountability. Now, the question is, accountability for what? For creating narrow, specific test scores? Or, for helping nourish better human beings? I have seen very little policy activities in the US – some in Asian countries such as Singapore and China – that are evaluating how to refine the curriculum for five to ten year olds. In the US, there was a major push for music enrichment programs in the late 90s that was somehow misguided. The problem is that although it is clear that enrichment has an impact it is tough to measure specifically what type of enrichment, since much of the benefit develops over time. The short-term "stock-market" mentality that measures student growth over a few weeks or months has to be tempered by long-term measures also.

For example, it seems clear that there are important skills that can be trained that make a better and more successful human being - such as the ability to defer gratification, sequencing, emotional intelligence, improved working memory, vocabulary, and processing skills. However, the type of assessments used today to measure school performance does not focus on these skills. We would need broader assessments to allow educators to focus on those important long-term skills, beyond the immediate pressures.

A specific area going from bad to worse is the level of stress in the system, and the lack of resources and knowledge to regulate it.

You mention processing skills, as well as other cognitive skills. In your recent column you highlight Scientific Learning's computer program (see Chapter 4 for more details on this program) that can train auditory processing. What is your view on the role of computer-based programs?

It is encouraging to see programs based on extensive research, such as Scientific Learning's. I appreciate the value of such programs to tailor individualized interventions to the needs of specific kids. So I believe these programs present a huge potential.

Now, we must not confuse what is just one narrow tool with a whole enrichment program. Brain-based education also must take into account other important factors such as nutrition, physical exercise, the arts, stress management, social interactions...I summarize much of this in my recent Phi Delta Kappa article.

Tell us more about interesting brain fitness research going on today.

The great news is that an increasing number of researchers are working with educators to find the best ways to bridge theory and practice. For example, UC Davis' Silvia Bunge is working with schools to measure the impact of cognitive training interventions not just on cognitive functions but also on how those benefits transfer to daily life. Researchers such as Larry Parsons are evaluating what type of music can enhance cognitive and academic performance.

What will have a larger and more sustained impact is the effort by the US National Institute of Health (NIH) to fund practical research done in a systematic manner. There is an ongoing initiative funded by the US National Science Foundation (NSF) that gathers thirty neuroscientists, including Scientific Learning's Paula Tallal who is part of the Temporal Dynamics Learning Center. This NSF program is designed to advance an integrated understanding of the role of time and timing in learning. The initiative has two corporate partners, Scientific Learning and Jensen Learning (our company).

In our conferences and workshops, we strive to make this emerging research meaningful for educators who want to improve their teaching. For example, educators are among the professions that should really know how to cope with chronic stress, given the growing research on how chronic stress affects neurogenesis and cognitive performance overall.

This is a stimulating and evolving field. What are some good online resources for educators who want to be informed about the latest developments and how these may influence their thinking and practices?

www.sciencedaily.com provides a continuous stream of fascinating news. Now, given that the amount of findings and news can be overwhelming, educators need to find "translators" they can trust, who analyze them and make them relevant. That's what my organization's conference tries to do twice a year. We aim to summarize the most important developments. It is also what Bob Sylwester has been doing in his Brain Connection monthly column or what our conferences aim to do. And what your SharpBrains team does as well - from a broader brain health perspective.

Interview with Dr. Robert Sylwester – Brain development.

BACKGROUND:

Dr. Robert Sylwester is an educator of educators. He has received multiple awards during his long career as a master communicator of the implications of brain science research for education and learning. He is the author of several books and many journal articles, and member of SharpBrains Scientific Advisory Board. His most recent book is *The Adolescent Brain: Reaching for Autonomy* (2007). He is an Emeritus Professor of Education at the University of Oregon.

HIGHLIGHTS:

- Significant human brain development happens after birth: Humans are born with an immature brain that develops mass and capabilities during 20 year after birth.
- Our brains are plastic: Every experience alters our brain's organization at some level.

LEARNING AND COGNITION

Let us start by defining some words such as learning, education, brain development and cognition.

Most organisms begin life with all of the processing systems and information that they need to survive. Humans are a notable exception in that an adult-size brain is significantly larger than a mother's birth canal. So, we are born with an immature one pound brain that develops additional mass and capabilities during its twenty year post-birth developmental trajectory. Parenting, mentoring, teaching, and mass media are examples of the cultural systems that humans have developed to help young people master the knowledge and skills they need to survive and thrive in complex environments. Learning is one of the main activities we do, even if many times we are not aware of it.

Education, like the culture it subsumes, is a conservative phenomenon. Science and technology move rapidly, education does not. So if schools often resemble the schools of fifty years ago, that should not be surprising. Parents remember their school experiences, and since they survived them, they are typically leery about educators "experimenting" with their children. Which explains why, in general, schools have not incorporated many of the lessons from neuroscience and cognitive psychology.

Childhood brain development is focused on systems that allow children to recognize and remember the dynamics of environmental challenges – challenges that protective adults will solve for them. Adolescent brain development is more focused on frontal lobe development, the systems that allow us to respond appropriately and autonomously to the challenges we confront.

Every remembered experience will alter our brain's organization at some level. Our brain's processing networks continually change throughout our life – this process is called brain plasticity. For example, my brain has adapted to my switch from using a typewriter to using a computer. So, it would now be difficult for me to relearn how to write on a typewriter.

Emotion is the system that tells us how important something is. Attention focuses us on the important and away from the unimportant things. Cognition tells us what to do about it. Cognitive skills are whatever it takes to do those things.

ROLE OF NATURE VS. NURTURE IN BRAIN DEVELOPMENT

What are the respective roles of genes and our environment in brain development?

Genetic and environmental factors both contribute to brain maturation. Genetics probably play a stronger role in the early years, and the environment plays a stronger role in later years. Still development can be affected by the mother's use of drugs during a pregnancy (this is an environmental factor). Some adult illnesses, such as Huntington's Disease, are genetically triggered.

We typically think of environmental factors as things that happen to us, over which we have little control. Can our own decisions have an effect in our own brain development? For example, what if I choose a career in investment banking, vs. one in journalism?

When we make our career decisions in life, most of us make a combination of good and bad decisions which have an influence on our brain maturation and development. My father was very unusual in his career trajectory in that he worked at one place throughout his entire adult life, and died three months after he retired at ninety-one years old. I have always thought that it is a good idea to make a change every ten years or so and do something different – either within the same organization or to move to another one. It is just as good for organizations to have some staff turnover as it is for staff to move to new challenges. The time to leave one position for another is while you and your employer are still happy with what you are doing.

You recently published a book titled The Adolescent Brain. What advice would you give to parents and educators of adolescents?

Biological phenomena always operate within ranges. For example, leaves fall from trees in the autumn, but not all at once. Developmental changes similarly do not all occur at the same time and at the same rate in every child and adolescent brain. And just as it is possible for wind or temperature to alter the time when a leaf might fall, unexpected events can alter the time when an adolescent has to confront and respond to given environmental challenges. The important thing for adults to do is to carefully observe an adolescent's interests and abilities, and insert challenges that move maturation forward at a reasonable level. If you push too fast, you end up with a stressed out adolescent. If you do not challenge sufficiently, you end up with a bored adolescent. No magic formula exists for getting this just right. This means, for example, that we celebrate the skills of artists and athletes who function beyond typical human capacity, and we create judicial sanctions for those whose behavior does not reach culturally acceptable levels. Most human behavior is personally chosen and executed within wide ranges. We can easily observe this wide range in such phenomena as political discourse and religious belief or practice. Adolescents strive towards autonomous adulthood as they gradually discover their interests and capabilities, and what is biologically possible and culturally appropriate. They adapt their life to wherever they're most comfortable within the marvelous sets of possible and appropriate ranges that exist.

Adolescents take risks, no doubt about that. If you want to eventually function within any range, you have to locate its outer positive and negative limits. Speed limits and other regulations provide direction, but adolescents (and adults) still tend to move towards the limits – and maybe just a smidge beyond. Bad things can then occur. Parents and educators need to pay attention to observe where adolescents' interests and abilities lie and actively engage them with experiences that will enable them to move forward.

There is a constant debate in education on whether we should focus efforts on nurturing all of the so-called "multiple intelligences," as defined by Howard Gardner, or focus on our strengths. What is your opinion?

Let me know when you have figured out the correct answer to this conundrum and I will contact the folks in Stockholm who give out the Nobel Prizes.

BRAIN RESOURCES

What are the most exciting areas of brain research, and what are some resources such as websites or books for educators to learn about the brain to refine their teaching?

The cognitive neurosciences are currently so dynamic that it seems like an exciting new development occurs every day, and many of these new developments are reported in the mass media. I write a monthly non-technical column on educationally significant developments in the cognitive neurosciences for the Internet journal Brain Connection. www.Sharpbrains.com is another great resource.

Interview with Lee Woodruff –
Recovering from traumatic brain injury.

BACKGROUND:

Bob Woodruff is a reporter who suffered a severe traumatic brain injury when a roadside bomb detonated next to his vehicle as he was covering news developments in Iraq. Lee Woodruff is Bob's wife and pillar throughout his spectacular recovery. Lee and Bob co-wrote the fantastic book *In an Instant: A Family's Journey of Love and Healing.*

HIGHLIGHTS:

- Chances for recovery after traumatic brain injury increase for people who have had an intellectually stimulating and diverse life.
- Cognitive therapy allows ones to recover by training the brain areas most damaged using challenging tasks that stimulate these areas.

Lee, many thanks for your time. I was amazed reading your book, where you share your journey, and then watching Bob interview John Edwards, the best display I can imagine of his recovery. Can you please summarize for us what Bob -and you- went through since January 2006?

As you know, Bob suffered a life-threatening traumatic brain injury in Iraq. He was promptly taken under military care and underwent a series of surgeries for head injuries, with a joint Army & Air Force neurosurgical team in Iraq, in a US Army Medical Command hospital in Germany, and at Bethesda Naval Hospital, back here in the US.

During this time, spanning around 4 months, he spent 37 days in coma, and his skull had to be surgically rebuilt. The cognitive rehabilitation process started then, at a medical facility closer home.

Can you please explain what kind of cognitive rehab Bob has gone though -both in a formal way, with a therapist, and informally, on his own?

The first thing I'd like to say is that rehab is a long process. Doctors told me that Bob, despite the severity of his injuries, had better chances to recover than other victims, because of the reserve of neurons and connections he had built thanks to an intellectually stimulating and diverse life, including living in China for several years and traveling to dozens of countries, having worked as a lawyer and as a journalist, and his overall curiosity and desire to learn. It seems that more and more research shows how people who are mentally active throughout their lives, either through their jobs, or doing puzzles, sudokus...are, of course up to a point, better prepared to deal with problems such as TBI.

Still, recovery is a long process. Bob had six months of structured cognitive therapy focused on speech and languages areas, because that was the part of his brain that had been most damaged. The therapist identified the main tasks for him to work on in a challenging, yet familiar way, usually asking Bob, for example, to read the New York Times, then try to remember what he had read, and write a short essay on his thoughts and impressions.

Since then he has, in a sense, used his work in the documentary To Iraq and Back and other projects at ABC as his informal, but very effective, way to keep improving. I am amazed to watch in real time how, even today, he gets better and better. To give you an example of his motivation to recover: he recently took on Chinese lessons to see if working on that also helped him.

In the book, Bob says that, if he had to say in one word what he was experiencing during much of the recovery, he would use the word "slower". His brain was slower at processing new information, at remembering words. What progress has he experienced?

A lot. He is not exactly at the same level he was before the injury, but he is again an amazing reporter, father, and husband. And I see progress every month, so we have hope that he will continue getting better and better.

Sometimes Bob tells me he is not the person I married. And then, as I mention in the book, I laugh and reply "I am not either. I'm older, wiser and more wrinkled."

I have learned to trust him. Especially in the beginning, it wasn't always easy to fully accept and follow his judgment, but I have seen how little by little he grew perfectly able to recreate his role as a husband and as a father, and to recreate our respective roles in the family. It has been wonderful to see that happen. It has been a miracle.

Bob has been a very fortunate survivor of traumatic brain injury. There are over a million cases of TBI every year. Many of them are military-related (a recent RAND study estimates that over 300,000 US service members have sustained TBI during assignments in Iraq or Afghanistan), but also happen in civilian life, mainly due to traffic accidents or sports concussions. What do we know today about how to prevent and treat TBI?

The Iraq War is literally re-writing the book, the way researchers and doctors see and tackle the problem. Most of the progress is happening in the military, but I hope that transfers into benefits for civilians, too. From a preventive point of view, the military has been stepping up to improve the body armor of soldiers, and I can now see why wearing seat belts as we drive and helmets as we bike can make a big difference.

From the recovery point of view, there is much more optimism and hope today than only a few years ago about how many TBI patients can improve, if given the opportunity to, through a supportive environment and physical and cognitive therapy. The military has recognized the problem of the so-called "Walking Wounded', and is devoting significant resources to analyzing best options and treating them. As we chatted earlier, the Army recently announced that from now on soldiers will get a cognitive screening before they get deployed to the field, so that in case there are problems that screening can serve as a good baseline to compare functions to.

But the improvement in the area is only starting. We need to see much progress.

Can you now tell us more about the Bob Woodruff Foundation for Traumatic Brain Injury? What are your main priorities?

Bob and I are devoting much time to raising awareness of the problem and the need to find and implement good solutions for cognitive care. Our foundation supports community, grass-roots approaches to helping TBI survivors and their families. Given the huge scale of the problem among the military, and the fact that Bob survived thanks to the excellent care he received from the military along the way, we are focusing first on helping military victims.

For example, we recently funded four scholarships for TBI-related research, and also bought 300 mattresses for a small non-profit that helps patients and their spouses rebuild their lives once they have to leave Army bases-many of whom cannot afford to move all their belongings, including beds and mattresses, out of the bases.

And there are many more things to do. For example, while many more soldiers are getting better care, that is not always the case with National Guard reservists who, despite having a dedicated branch of the armed forces oversee their progress, are often more at risk of living with undetected TBI since they don't have to report to bases once they are back.

It is also not clear that the military (as well as insurance companies) are always willing to pay for the long-term costs of care.

What are some specific ways people can support the work of your foundation?

They can visit our new website, Bob Woodruff Foundation (http://remind. org/), to learn about the problems and to donate funds, no matter how big or small. We are also holding a fundraising event in NYC in November to raise awareness.

But probably the most important thing every one can do is to recognize the sacrifices the soldiers have made, and find active ways to look for them and help them in their own communities. Soldiers and their families often have grown up in a culture of self-reliance, of not asking for help, so here we all need to take the initiative to figure out how we can help. Ask yourself, how can I help the TBI survivors in my neighborhood? Perhaps by giving them a job, or offering them help or training, so they can secure one? How can I help their spouses and families maintain healthy and happy environments? Perhaps by offering them free movie tickets? A massage?

Lee, many thanks for those suggestions. I do have friends at a local Veteran Affairs hospital, and will follow-up on those great ideas. I hope our readers can also think of ways they can help (and exercise their brains along the way). Is there something else you would like to add, that you would like everyone to be aware of?

I'd say never give up. We have seen how Bob has recovered, which I think is a miracle. Let's simply try our best to help everyone out there.

Chapter 2.

The 4 Pillars of Brain Maintenance

HIGHLIGHTS

- Thanks to lifelong neuroplasticity and neurogenesis, our lifestyles and actions play a meaningful role in how our brains physically change.
- There is no "general solution" to brain maintenance. A multi-pronged approach centered on nutrition, stress management, and both physical and mental exercise is recommended for better brain health.

In Chapter 1 you learned about brain functions and neuroplasticity. As you will discover in the present chapter, the idea of brain maintenance rests upon these two key concepts. Before focusing on brain training in Chapter 3 we would like to give you now an overall view of what one can do to maintain good brain health.

2.1. WHY YOUR LIFESTYLE MATTERS

The latest scientific research shows that specific lifestyles and actions can, no matter our age, improve the health and level of functioning of our brains. Such improvement can happen thanks to neuroplasticity that is, when the rate of creation and survival of new neurons in certain parts of the brain is increased, or when the rate of creation and survival of synapses (the connections between neurons) speeds up, or when a neurochemical environment is nurtured in our brains to support information processing.

The nice thing about discovering that our lifestyle can affect brain functions is that it puts our brain health largely under our own control. However there is no magic formula. Scientists are only beginning to understand how what we do can interact with our genetic makeup. As to now, it is not possible to define which actions are the best for which individuals. It is likely that there will never be one general solution that solves all the challenges inherent in maintaining one's brain health. Dr. Art Kramer, whose interview can be found at the end of this Chapter, points out that a multitude of approaches will be necessary.

So what factors have an influence on brain health?

Current recommendations suggest that a brain-healthy life style should include at least balanced nutrition, stress management, physical exercise, and brain exercise. Other factors may also have an influence. Dr. Elizabeth Zelinski, whose interview can be found at the end of the present Chapter, points out that "it is also important to maintain emotional connections. Not only with ourselves, to have self-confidence and self-esteem, but also with our family our friends." Sleep and overall health conditions are other factors that also matter.

Here we focus on the four main pillars of brain health:

- Balanced nutrition
- Stress management
- Physical exercise
- Mental stimulation

2.2. PILLAR 1: NUTRITION GUIDELINES

How can nutrition influence brain functions?

First of all, the brain consumes a considerable amount of glucose. One of the earliest sign of dementia is a decrease in the ability of the brain to use glucose efficiently. As such a dysfunction is at the core of diabetes, some neuroscientists refer to Alzheimer's Disease as Type 3 diabetes.

The brain is also a fatty organ. Fats are present in the neurons' membranes to keep them flexible. These fats are the omega 3 and omega 6 fatty acids molecules. Our brain is dependent on dietary fat intake to get enough fatty acids. Omega-3 fatty acids can be found in cold-water fish (such as mackerel, herring, salmon, and tuna), kiwi, and walnuts. Docosahexaenoic acid, or DHA, is the most abundant omega-3 fatty acid in cell membranes in the brain.

In general, the brain is highly susceptible to oxidative damage. This is why antioxidant food has become popular for their positive effects on brain function. Antioxidants are found in a variety of food: Alpha lipoic is found in spinach, broccoli and potatoes; Vitamin E is found in vegetable oils, nuts, green leafy vegetables; Vitamin C is found in citrus fruit and several plants and vegetables. Berries are well known for their antioxidant capacity but it is not clear which of their many components has an effect on cognition.

Based on these observations, Dr. Larry McCleary (whose interview you will find at the end of this Chapter) recommends a diet containing fatty fish, vegetables and salads, non-starchy fruits (like berries) - that are high in free radical fighting compounds - and nuts.

As most people you probably have bought or thought of buying nutrition complements. Indeed it is hard to get all the good nutrients in one's diet. The most common consumer purchase is herbal and vitamin supplements purported to improve memory. Table 2 shows you the most recent findings associated with well-known supplements such as Ginkgo biloba.

However one has to be cautious. One negative aspect of self-medication with herbal supplements is the fact that some products have been shown to counteract the effects of prescription and over-the-counter medications. For example, in 2001, Dr. Piscitelli from the National Institute of Health (NIH) showed a significant drug interaction between St. John's wort (hypericum perforatum), an herbal product sold as a dietary supplement, and Indinavir, a protease inhibitor used to treat HIV infection. The herb has also caused negative interactions with cancer chemotherapeutic drugs and with birth control drugs.

Experts usually recommend a balanced diet, that is getting healthy nutrients (Omega-3, antioxidants, etc.) from the food you eat, rather than ingesting supplements. Few studies so far have shown that supplements are beneficial to brain health. More importantly the best dosage of these supplements is not known.

SUPPLEMENT	RECENT EVIDENCE
DHEA A steroid precursor to testosterone and estrogen purported to fight aging.	The conclusion of a two-year study at the Mayo Clinic in Minnesota and University of Padua in Italy showed that DHEA did not improve strength, physical performance, or other measures of health. The study's lead author, Dr. Nair (2006) said, "No beneficial effects on quality of life were observed. There's no evidence based on this study that DHEA has an anti-aging effect."
Ginkgo biloba An over-the-counter "memory-enhancing" supplement.	In 2002 Dr. Paul Solomon from Williams College found that "when taken following the manufacturer's instructions, ginkgo provides no measurable benefit in memory or related cognitive function to adults with healthy cognitive function." Dr. Burns (2006) from the University of Adelaide, Australia found longer-term memory improved in healthy fifty-five to seventy-nine year olds, but no other cognitive measure improved for younger participants. Dr. Elsabagh (2005) from King's College London found that ginkgo initially improved attention and memory. However, there were no benefits after 6 weeks, suggesting that a tolerance develops quickly. A recent randomized trial (DeKosky et al., 2008), conducted in 5 academic medical centers in the United States and including 2587 volunteers aged 75 years or older with normal cognition, showed that G biloba at 120 mg twice a day was not effective in reducing the overall incidence rate of dementia.
Omega-3 fatty acids Components of neurons' membranes.	Dr. Fontani's work at the University of Siena in Italy associated omega-3 supplementation with improved attentional and physiological functions, particularly those involving complex cortical processing.

TABLE 2. Summary of recent findings on supposedly brain-enhancing dietary supplements.

2.3. PILLAR 2: STRESS MANAGEMENT

Prolonged exposure to high levels of stress can damage the brain. As part of a brain-healthy life-style it is essential to manage stress efficiently.

It is clear that our society has changed more rapidly than our genes have. Today, instead of being faced with physically and immediately life-threatening crises that demand instant action, we more regularly deal with events and illnesses that gnaw away at us slowly without any stress release.

In his book, *Why Zebras don't have Ulcers*, Dr. Sapolsky points out that humans are unique in that they are the only mammals who can get stressed from their own thoughts. When humans are stressed, for any reason, they have the same kind of stress reaction that, for example, a zebra would when it tries to escape from the clutches of a lion. However, in trying to save its life by running away, the zebra essentially uses up its stress hormones to fuel its escape. Humans, on the other hand, usually just keep muddling along and let the stress build up over long periods of time.

Overall, stress limits mental flexibility and one's ability to see alternative solutions. As such, it can prevent us from adapting to, and succeeding in, new circumstances. It can also lead to various cardiac and immune problems. Although stress is an unavoidable consequence of modern life, when work stress becomes too much, it can lead to burnout.

Prolonged exposure to adrenal steroid hormones like cortisol, which is released into the blood stream when we are stressed, can damage the brain and block the formation of new neurons in the hippocampus, the key actor in encoding new memories in the brain. Chronic stress leads to cell death and hampers our ability to make changes and be creative enough to think of possible changes we could make to reduce the stress.

General Adaptation Syndrome (GAS) describes the long-term, nasty kind of stress that does not go away. This is the kind of stress that paralyzes someone into inaction. The common reaction to this type of stress is to think about a problem and worry about it without doing anything about it. This is the kind of stress that kills neurons, destroys immune and cardiovascular systems, and makes a person anxious, irritable, and unable to sleep.

What can you do once you have realized that you are stressed? As you can see in Table 3, the best defenses against chronic stress are physical exercise, relaxation, self-empowerment, and cultivating social networks. Biofeedback has also been mentioned as useful in stress reduction. As an example, in 1998, a study showed that self-management programs using techniques designed to eliminate negative thought loops and promote positive emotional states can successfully decrease cortisol levels (McCraty and colleagues, 1998).

How to manage stress	
Exercise	Exercise can reduce the experience of stress, depression, and anxiety.
Relax	Relaxation, whether through meditation, tai chi, yoga or taking a walk by the beach, lowers blood pressure, slows respiration and metabolism and releases muscle tension.
Socialize	Cultivating social networks of friends, family and even pets can help foster trust, support and also relaxation.
Empower yourself	Finding ways to empower oneself can be a defense against chronic stress since self-confidence and taking control of one's environment helps to resolve the stress response.
Use biofeedback programs	Biofeedback program (see Chapter 3) that generate real-time information on stress levels can provide a unique opportunity to learn effective techniques for reducing stress levels.

TABLE 3. A few solutions to deal with chronic stress. Chronic stress can damage the brain and thus impair brain functions.

Is stress always bad? There is such thing as "positive" stress. This stress is often experienced as butterflies in the stomach or sweaty palms felt before a big athletic game, artistic performance or speech. The same stress may also surface at work before a presentation or important phone call or meeting. This "positive" stress may boost performance as cortisol usually combines with adrenaline in such circumstances. However, this kind of stress is short lived. The adrenaline is evident for a period of time and then it gets essentially used up as the goal is accomplished. And, once the goal is accomplished, there is typically time to rest and recover while basking in the glow of having completed the task.

2.4. PILLAR 3: PHYSICAL EXERCISE

As little as three hours a week of brisk walking has been shown to halt, and even reverse, the brain atrophy (shrinkage) that starts in a person's forties, especially in the regions responsible for memory and higher cognition. Exercise increases the brain's volume of gray matter (actual neurons) and white matter (connections between neurons).

Through increased blood flow to the brain, physical exercise triggers biochemical changes that spur neuroplasticity – the production of new connections between neurons and even of neurons themselves. Brain exercise then protects these fledgling neurons by bathing them in a nerve growth factor and forming functional connections with neighboring neurons. Dr. Gage's work of the Salk Institute for Biological Studies, have shown that exercise helps generate new brain cells, even in the aging brain.

Studying this topic, Dr. Smeyne of the Saint Jude Children's Research Hospital in Memphis, found that results could be seen in two months in Parkinson patients. Parkinson patients demonstrate a progressive loss of dopamine neurons in the substantia nigra pars. After two months of exercise, the patients had more brain cells. Higher levels of exercise were shown to be significantly more beneficial than lower amounts, although any exercise was better than none. Smeyne also found that starting an exercise program early in life was an effective way to lower the risk of developing Parkinson's disease later in life.

Numerous animal studies have shown that physical exercise has a multitude of effects on the brain beyond neurogenesis, including increases in various neurotransmitters and nerve growth factor levels, and angiogenesis (the formation of new blood vessels).

In 2003, Dr. Colcombe and Kramer, analyzed the results of 18 scientific studies published between 2000 and 2001. The results of this meta-analysis clearly showed that physical fitness training increases cognitive performance in healthy adults between the ages of 55 and 80.

Another meta-analysis published in 2004 by Dr. Heyn and colleagues shows similar beneficial effects of fitness training for people over 65 years old who had cognitive impairment or dementia.

What type of exercises is needed?

According to Dr. Art Kramer, aerobic exercise, at least thirty to sixty minutes per day, three days a week, has been shown to have a positive impact on brain functions. Importantly, the exercise does not have to be strenuous, walking have been shown to have positive effects too.

2.5. PILLAR 4: MENTAL STIMULATION

The cognitive or brain reserve hypothesis states that it is possible to build up the brain's resilience to neuronal damage and delay the onset of Alzheimer's symptoms. The concept of brain reserve stems from the repeated observation that the relationship between clinical symptoms and actual brain pathology is not direct. For example, Katzman and colleagues (1989) described 10 cases of cognitively normal older adults who, at death, were discovered to have advanced Alzheimer's disease pathology in their brains. The researchers hypothesized that these individuals did not show symptoms of Alzheimer's because they had larger brains, that is more neurons. The idea is that having a larger "reserve" of neurons and abilities can offset the losses caused by Alzheimer's. The concept of cognitive/brain reserve is thus defined as the ability of an individual to tolerate progressive brain pathology (including Alzheimer's plaques and tangles) without demonstrating clinical cognitive symptoms.

Subsequent research has shown that frequent participation in mentally stimulating activities reduces the risk of Alzheimer's disease, possibly by increasing brain reserve. As a consequence, brain activity or exercise in general is hypothesized to help increase brain reserve.

In our view, brain training is more than the stimulation triggered by challenging daily activities. We define brain training as the structured use of cognitive exercises aimed at improving specific brain functions (see Chapter 3).

Rigorous and targeted brain training has been used in clinical practice for many years as a way of helping patients recovering from the effects of traumatic brain injury, stroke, and other neurological disorders. It can help improve memory, attention, confidence and competence, reasoning skills, and even reduce anxiety.

Past research outside the clinical domain has shown that cognitive abilities can also be trained systematically in healthy individuals. Individuals trained in a specific task usually will become better at this task (see for instance Willis et al., 2006 or Ball et al., 2002). What is even more important, such training sometimes has generalized effects improving performance on other, similar tasks.

Although it has been long thought that "you cannot teach old dogs new tricks", many studies show that cognition can be trained at all ages. In particular, many studies have shown that middle age individuals as well as older individuals can learn techniques to boost their memory (see for example Brooks et al., 1999; Derwinger et al., 2003 or the meta-analysis published by Verhaeghen et al. in 1992).

If we could summarize a variety of research fields and findings into a few useful guidelines, we would say that "good" brain exercise requires variety, challenge and novelty. These guidelines are described in Table 4.

Varied, novel and challenging exercises will necessarily induce learning. Learning is critical. When one learns a new fact or a new way of accomplishing a task, neurons and synapses – connections – in the brain change. This is neuroplasticity as defined early. The changes associated with learning may help increase one's brain reserve, contributing to general brain health.

Learning and changing is never easy. This requires effort. As Dr. James Zull points out learning and changing require getting out of our comfort zones. Often, the fear of failing is a key obstacle to learning.

Recipe for a good mental exercise	
Variety	Excessive specialization is not the best strategy for long-term brain health. A better strategy is to stimulate the multiple functions of the brain. This can be done by creating a mental "workout circuit" similar to a physical exercise circuit in a health club since our brains are composed of multiple structures with multiple functions.
Challenge	The goal is to be exposed to increasing levels of challenge, so that a task never becomes too easy or routine.
Novelty	Trying new things is important since very important parts of the brain, such as the prefrontal cortex, are mostly exercised when we learn to master new cognitive challenges.

TABLE 4. The recipe for a good mental exercise

2.6. BRAIN MAINTENANCE: ALZHEIMER'S PREVENTION OR COGNITIVE ENHANCEMENT?

Brain maintenance may play a role in postponing the emergence of dementia-related symptoms. A significant amount of research has been conducted on healthy aging in the past two decades. A number of factors have been associated with reduced risks of developing Alzheimer's disease.

Among these factors, mental activities range quite high. As we described earlier, people who remain intellectually active and engaged in hobbies throughout their lives reduce their risk of developing Alzheimer's disease and other dementias. In a 2001 study conducted by Dr. Yaakov Stern, leading researcher on the cognitive reserve, individuals with the highest level of leisure activities presented thirty-eight percent less risk (controlling for other factors) of developing Alzheimer's symptoms. For each additional type of activity, the risks were reduced by eight percent. It is believed that intellectually stimulating hobbies or activities help building up cognitive reserve. This can help postponing the appearance of the dementia's symptoms.

Interestingly, education also seems to have a protective effect. Research into cognitive reserve found that the more education people have, the less they suffer from age-related decline. High levels of education have also been associated with lower risks levels for Alzheimer's disease (Snowdon et al., 1989; Wilson et al., 2002). It is possible that the effect of education is related to the effects of intellectual stimulation as well-educated people are more likely to have cognitively stimulating jobs.

According to Dr. Arthur Kramer (whose interview you can find at the end of this chapter) the two key lifestyle habits that may help someone delay Alzheimer's symptoms and improve overall brain health are to stay physically active and to maintain lifelong intellectual engagement. However, no specific program has been shown to prevent Alzheimer's disease completely.

In sum, brain maintenance in general can be viewed as a way of preventing cognitive declines associated with aging and dementia to occur too early. Note however that, as Dr. Jerri Edwards (whose interview you can find at the end of Chapter 5) points out, it is too early to say whether we can really reverse decline in a permanent way. Brain functions are complex and well-conducted studies looking at the long-term effects of brain exercises are yet to be conducted.

What about brain training itself? As we have explained in this chapter, brain maintenance is more than intellectual stimulation or more than brain exercise. We defined brain training as the structured use of cognitive exercises aimed at improving specific brain functions. In this view, preventing Alzheimer's is not the main or only premise (or objective) of brain training. Rather, improving quality of life and cognitive performance is. The same as one goes to a health club and engages in a workout circuit to improve physical abilities, brain training can be viewed as a "mental workout" to help maintain a variety of cognitive abilities.

2.7. BRAIN MAINTENANCE: SUMMARY AND GUIDELINES

– *Balanced nutrition*: As a general guideline, what is good for the body is also good for the brain. Eating a variety of foods of different colors including cold-water fish which contain omega-3 fatty acids and avoiding highly processed foods with added ingredients are recommended. Vegetables, particularly green, leafy ones, are also recommended whereas few well known supplements have shown long-term benefits on memory and other cognitive functions.

- *Stress management*: Chronic stress reduces and can even inhibit neurogenesis. Meditation, yoga, and other calming activities are effective in countering stress. Biofeedback devices that measure heart rate variability and show stress levels in real-time offer a more high-tech option to manage stress.
- *Physical exercise*: Physical exercise has been shown to enhance brain physiology in animals and, more recently, in humans. Physical exercise improves learning through increased blood supply and growth hormone levels in the body. Of all the types of physical exercise, cardiovascular exercise that gets the heart beating – from walking to skiing, tennis and basketball – has been shown to have the greatest effect.
- *Mental stimulation*: it strengthens the synapses or connections between neurons, thus improving neuron survival and cognitive functioning. Good mental exercise requires novelty, variety and increasing levels of challenge.

Important take-away: these pillars are complementary, they do not substitute each other. It is important for a person to recognize their starting point, and identify what pillar they may need to focus more on.

For each pillar or lifestyle factor, it is important to be creative in finding a schedule or routine that works for an individual through trial and error.

According to Dr. Art Kramer, the ideal way would be to combine physical and mental stimulation along with social interaction: "Why not take a good walk with friends to discuss a book? We all lead very busy lives, so the more integrated and interesting our activities are, the more likely we will engage in them."

Now, what can you do to start your healthy-brain lifestyle tomorrow? Have a look at Table 5 for several lifestyle tips that are easy to implement.

How to live a brain-healthy lifestyle	
Balanced Nutrition	• Eat a variety of foods of different colors without a lot of added ingredients or processes. • Plan your meals around your vegetables, and then add fruit, protein, dairy, and/or grains. • Add some cold-water fish to your diet (tuna, salmon, mackerel, halibut, sardines, and herring), which contain omega-3 fatty acids. • Go to the United States Department of Agriculture website at www.mypyramid.gov to learn what a portion-size is, so you don't overeat. • Try to eat more foods low on the Glycemic Index (learn more at www.glycemicindex.com). • If you can only do one thing, eat more vegetables, particularly leafy green ones.
Stress management	• Get regular cardiovascular exercise. • Try to get enough sleep each night (i.e. six to eight hours). • Stay connected with friends and family. • Practice meditation, yoga, or some other calming activity as a way to take a relaxing time-out. • Try training with a heart rate variability sensor, like the one in the emWave® Stress Management programs. • If you can only do one thing, set aside 5-10 minutes a day to just breathe deeply and recharge.

Physical Exercise	• Start by talking to your doctor, especially if you are not currently physically active, have special health concerns, or are making significant changes to your current program. • Set a goal that you can achieve. Do something you enjoy for even just 15 minutes a day; you can always add more time and variety later. • Schedule exercise into your daily routine. It will become a habit faster if you do. • If you can only do one thing, do something cardiovascular, i.e. something that gets your heart beating faster. This includes walking, running, skiing, swimming, biking, hiking, tennis, basketball, playing tag, ultimate Frisbee, and other similar sports/activities.
Mental Stimulation	• Do a variety of things, including things you are not good at for novelty (if you like to sing, try painting or dancing). • Be curious! Get to know your local library and community college, look for local organizations that offer classes and workshops, or join a book club. • Work puzzles like crosswords and sudoku or play games like chess and bridge. However, make sure to introduce novelty and variety – doing more of the same is not what helps most. • Try a computerized brain fitness program for a customized workout.

TABLE 5. Lifestyle tips that you may consider for each of the four pillars of brain health.

2.8. INTERVIEWS

- Dr. Yaakov Stern: The connection between building a cognitive reserve and delaying Alzheimer's symptoms.
- Dr. Larry McCleary: A multi-pronged approach to brain health.
- Dr. Arthur Kramer: Why we need both physical and mental exercise.
- Dr. Elizabeth Zelinski: Healthy aging enhanced with computer-based programs.

Interview with Dr. Yaakov Stern –
The connection between building a cognitive
reserve and delaying Alzheimer's symptoms.

BACKGROUND:

Dr. Stern is the Division Leader of the Cognitive Neuroscience Division of the Sergievsky Center, and Professor of clinical neuropsychology, at the College of Physicians and Surgeons of Columbia University, New York.

He is one of the leading proponents of the cognitive reserve theory, which aims to explain why some individuals with Alzheimer's pathology (accumulation of plaques and tangles in their brains) can keep normal lives until they die, while others with the same amount of plaques and tangles display the severe symptoms we associate with Alzheimer's Disease.

HIGHLIGHTS:

- A lifetime of engaging activities has a positive cumulative effect: Lifetime factors such as education, occupation, and activities, have a major influence on how we age. The more activities we do throughout our lives, the better.
- Stimulating activities, ideally combining physical exercise, learning and social interaction, help build a cognitive reserve to protect us. The earlier we start building our reserve, the better; but it is never too late to start.

DEFINING THE COGNITIVE RESERVE

The implications of your research are astounding, presenting major implications across sectors and age groups. What has been the most unexpected reaction you have received so far?

I was pretty surprised when, years ago, a reporter from *Seventeen* magazine requested an interview. I was really curious to learn why she felt that her readers would be interested in studies about dementia. What she told me showed a deep understanding and insight: she wanted to motivate children to stay in school and not drop out.

She understood that early social interventions could be very powerful for building a reserve and preventing dementia.

Fast forward 60 or so years from high-school. Suppose that two people A and B both technically have Alzheimer's (plaques and tangles appear in the brain), but only A is showing the disease symptoms. What may explain this discrepancy?

Individuals who lead mentally stimulating lives, through education, occupation and leisure activities, have reduced risk of developing Alzheimer's. Studies suggest that they have thirty-five to forty percent less risk of manifesting the disease. The pathology will still occur, but they are able to cope with it better. Some will not ever be diagnosed with Alzheimer's because they will not present any symptoms. In studies that follow healthy elders over time and then study their brains through autopsies, up to twenty percent of people who did not present any significant problem in the daily lives have full blown Alzheimer's pathology in their brains.

What is going on in the brain to provide that level of protection?

There are two ideas that are complementary. One idea (called brain reserve by researchers) postulates that some individuals have a greater number of neurons and synapses, and that somehow those extra structures provide a level of protection. In a sense, they have more "hardware", providing a passive protection against the attacks of Alzheimer's.

The other theory (called cognitive reserve) emphasizes the building of new capabilities, how people can perform tasks better through practice, and how these skills become so well learned that they are not easy to unlearn. It is like developing new and refined "software."

Both scenarios seem to go hand in hand, correct? Does neuroplasticity mean that what you call "hardware" and "software" are two sides of the same coin and they influence each other?

Correct. So these days we do not make a sharp distinction, and are conducting more neuroimaging studies to better understand the relationship between both.

BUILDING THE COGNITIVE RESERVE

If the goal is to build that cognitive reserve of neurons, synapses, and skills, how can we do that? What defines mentally stimulating activities or good brain exercise?

In summary, we could say that "brain stimulation" consists of engaging in activities. In our research almost all activities are seen to contribute to building the reserve. Some have challenging levels of cognitive complexity, and some have interpersonal or physical demands. In animal studies, exposure to an enriched environment or increased physical activity results in increased neurogenesis (the creation of new neurons). You can get that stimulation through education and/ or your occupation. There is clear research showing how those two elements reduce the risk.

What is very exciting is that, no matter one's age, education and occupation, our level of participation in leisure activities has a significant and cumulative effect. A key message here is that different activities have independent, synergistic effects. This means that the more things you do and the earlier you start, the better. But you are never stuck. It is better to start late than never.

Can you give us some examples of leisure activities that seem to have the most positive effects?

For our 2001 study we evaluated the effect of thirteen activities, combining intellectual, physical, and social elements. Some of the activities with the most effect were reading, visiting friends or relatives, going to movies or restaurants, and walking for pleasure or going on an excursion. As you can see, there are a variety of options.

We saw that the group with a high level of leisure activities presented thirty-eight percent less risk (controlling for other factors) of developing Alzheimer's symptoms. And that, for each additional type of activity, the risk got reduced by eight percent.

There is also an additional element that we are starting to see more clearly. Physical exercise, by itself, also has a very beneficial impact on cognition. Only a few months ago researchers were able to show for the first time how physical activity promotes neurogenesis in the human brain.

So, we need both mental and physical exercise. The not-so-good news is that, as of today, there is no clear recipe for success. More research is needed before we can prepare a systematic set of interventions that can help maximize our protection.

We often hear about the importance of good nutrition, physical exercise, stress management and mental exercise that present novelty, variety and challenge. What do you think of the relatively recent appearance of so many computer-based cognitive training programs, some more science-based than others?

The elements you mention make sense. The problem is that, at least from the point of view of Alzheimer's, we cannot be much more specific. We do not know if learning a new language is more beneficial than learning a new musical instrument or using a computer-based program.

A few of the cognitive training computer programs we have seen, like the one you discussed with Professor Daniel Gopher to train the mental abilities of pilots, seem to have clear effects on cognition, generalizing beyond the training itself. But, for the most part, it is too early to tell the long-term effects. We need better designed clinical trials with clear controls. Right now, the most we can say is that those who lead mentally stimulating lives, through education, occupation and leisure activities seem to have the least risk of developing Alzheimer's disease.

Interview with Dr. Larry McCleary – A multi-pronged approach to brain health.

BACKGROUND:

Dr. Larry McCleary is a former acting Chief of Pediatric Neurosurgery at Denver Children's Hospital and author of *The Brain Trust Program* (2007).

HIGHLIGHTS:

- Brain health requires a holistic approach involving appropriate nutrition, stimulating brain activities, physical activities, and stress reduction.
- No matter one's brain status or age, there is much one can do to improve brain functions.

BRAIN HEALTH IS AVAILABLE TO EVERYONE

As a neurosurgeon, how did you develop an interest in brain health public education?

For two reasons: I am a Baby Boomer and am trying to maximize my own brain health. Also, there is a great deal of exciting research documenting how we can be proactive in this regard. This information needs to be disseminated and I would like to help in this process.

And what is the single most important brain-related idea or concept that you would like every person in the planet to fully understand?

The most important take home message about brain health is that we now know that no matter what your brain status or age, there is much you can do to significantly improve brain functions and slow brain aging. Based on emerging information, what is especially nice is the fact that unlike many things in life our brain health is largely under own control.

NOURISHING OUR BRAINS

What are the most important elements to nourish our brains as we age?

I approach this question much like how an athlete prepares for a competition. Professional athletes use a holistic approach. This is also what a healthy brain requires. It should not be surprising that "what is good for the body is good for the brain." That is how our bodies and brains evolved.

Hence what I believe are valuable components of a well-rounded approach to brain health are appropriate nutrition, stimulating brain activities, physical activities, and stress reduction.

How can we nourish our brains?

The major fuel the brain consumes is glucose. The earliest sign of impending dementia and Alzheimer Disease (AD) is a decrease in the ability of the brain to use glucose efficiently. Based on this observation, some neuroscientists are referring to AD as Type 3 diabetes because of the inability to appropriately use glucose in that disorder. This makes sense because people with diabetes have a four-fold increase in AD.

The brain is a fatty organ. The most important fats are those in the nerve cell membranes whose presence keeps them flexible. These are the long chain omega 3 fatty acid molecules found in fatty, cold-water fish and arachidonic acid (a long chain omega 6 fatty acid). These are both delicate fats and as such can oxidize easily (meaning they can become rancid). Thus, we should include additional dietary components that provide free radical fighting activity to protect them against oxidation.

Based on these observations, I recommend a diet containing fatty fish, veggies and salads, non-starchy fruits (like berries) - that are high in free radical fighting compounds - and nuts.

PILLARS OF BRAIN HEALTH

What is the value of stimulating brain activity?

To increase neuroplasticity (the continual ability of the brain to "rewire" itself) and neurogenesis (the formation of new nerve cells), brain stimulation is vital. All types count including schoolwork, occupational endeavors, leisure activities and formal brain training. The key in any activity is to include novelty (to encourage thinking outside the box), challenge and variety.

And, physical activity?

Exercise delivers additional blood and oxygen to the brain. Yet, it does so much more. It actually causes alterations in the nerve cells. They produce more neurotrophins, which are compounds that increase the formation of new nerve cells and enhance their connectivity. They also make the neurons we have more resistant to the aging process. I recommend cross-training your brain by starting with a good aerobic program and mix in resistance (weight training) exercise and speed and agility components such as jumping rope, playing ping-pong, gymnastics and various balance drills.

How does stress reduction relate?

Chronic, unremitting stress kills neurons. This is especially detrimental to memory function. So include a component of stress reduction in your approach to optimal brain health and make sure to get plenty of sleep.

Also, be aware of the side effects of some medications. There are medications that lower the level of important brain nutrients in the body such as B vitamins and coenzyme Q10. Check with your doctor to screen for these. There are also many common medicines (many OTC) that have anti-cholinergic activities. These can impair the function of one of the most important memory neurotransmitters in the brain - acetylcholine.

ADVICE FOR HEALTH PROFESSIONALS

What brain health-related information or practices would you suggest to other doctors and health professionals, both for themselves and for the patients they see?

They should counsel their patients on tips for brain health such as those listed above in much the same way they discuss cardiac risk factors and how to address them. I would like to see physicians encourage their patients to avoid high-fructose corn syrup because it has recently been shown to be associated with increased brain atrophy.

Interview with Dr. Arthur Kramer – Why we need both physical and mental exercise.

BACKGROUND:

Dr. Arthur Kramer is a Professor in the Department of Psychology at the University of Illinois. At the University, he is part of the Campus Neuroscience Program, the Beckman Institute, and the Director of the Biomedical Imaging Center.

HIGHLIGHTS:

- Aerobic exercise, at least thirty to sixty minutes per day, three days a week, has an impact on brain fitness.
- The ideal for brain health: combine both physical and mental stimulation along with social interactions.

LIFESTYLE CHOICES TO ENHANCE BRAIN HEALTH

Let's start by trying to clarify some existing misconceptions and controversies. Based on what we know today, and your recent article in Nature, what are the top two or three key lifestyle habits that you suggest would help someone delay Alzheimer's symptoms and improve overall brain health?

First, be Active. Do physical exercise. Aerobic exercise, at least thirty to sixty minutes per day, three days a week, has been shown to have an impact in a variety of experiments. And you do not need to do something strenuous. Even walking has shown to have this effect. There are many open questions in terms of specific types of exercise, duration, and magnitude of effect. But, as we wrote in our recent Nature Reviews Neuroscience article, there is little doubt that leading a sedentary life is bad for our cognitive health. Cardiovascular exercise seems to have a positive effect.

Second, maintain lifelong intellectual engagement. There is abundant observational research showing that doing more mentally stimulating activities reduces the risk of developing Alzheimer's symptoms.

Ideally, combine both physical and mental stimulation along with social interactions. Why not take a good walk with friends to discuss a book? We all lead very busy lives, so the more integrated and interesting our activities are, the more likely we will do them.

Great concept: a walking book club! Part of the confusion we are seeing in the marketplace is due to the search for "the magic bullet" that will work for everyone and solve all problems. We prefer to talk about the four pillars of brain health and to focus on the different priorities for each individual. Can you elaborate on what interventions seem to have a positive effect on specific cognitive abilities, for specific individuals?

Perhaps one day we will be able to recommend specific interventions for individuals based on genetic testing, for example, but we do not have a clue today. We are only beginning to understand how the environment interacts with our genome. But, I agree with the premise that there probably will not be a general solution that solves all cognitive problems, but that we need a multitude of approaches. And we cannot forget, for example, the cognitive benefits from smoking cessation, sleep, pharmacological interventions, nutrition, and social engagement.

Physical exercise tends to have rather broad effects on different forms of perception and cognition, as seen in the Colcombe and Kramer, 2003, meta-analysis published in Psychological Science.

Cognitive training also works for a multitude of perceptual and cognitive domains – but has shown little transfer beyond trained tasks. No single type of intervention is sufficient. Today there is no clear research on how those different lifestyle factors may interact. The National Institute on Aging is starting to sponsor research to address precisely this question.

Earlier you said that no brain software in particular has been shown to maintain cognition across extended periods of time. Now, didn't the ACTIVE trial five-year results show how cognitive training (computerized or not) can result in pretty durable results? For context, are there comparable controlled studies to ACTIVE where ten or more hours of physical exercise today can result in measurable (yet, incomplete) cognitive benefits five years from now?

The ACTIVE study showed a good deal of five years retention of the tasks that were trained for ten hours each, but limited transfer of training was found for other untrained tasks. It seems unlikely that significant transfer may occur with the relatively little training (e.g. ten hours in the ACTIVE study) and focused tasks that have been provided in training studies thus far.

On whether there are controlled studies similar to ACTIVE that have measured the long-term cognitive benefits of physical exercise, there are none that I know of.

What is the best way to explain the relative benefits of physical vs. cognitive exercise? It seems clear that physical exercise can help enhance neurogenesis (i.e. the creation of new neurons), yet learning and cognitive exercise contribute to the survival of those neurons by strengthening synapses, so it seems that those two "pillars" are more complementary than interchangeable.

I agree. Given what we know today, I would recommend both intellectual engagement and physical exercise. However, we do know, from a multitude of animal studies, that physical exercise has a multitude of effects on brains beyond neurogenesis, including increases in various neurotransmitters, nerve growth factors, and angiogenesis (the formation of new blood vessels).

FLEXIBILITY OF SENIORS' BRAINS

Tell us more about your work with cognitive training for older adults.

We now have a study in press where we evaluate the effect of a commercially available strategy videogame on older adults' cognition (Note: this study is now published, see Basak, et al., 2008)

Let me first give some context. It seems clear that, as we age, our so-called crystallized abilities remain pretty stable, whereas the so-called fluid abilities decline. One particular set of fluid abilities is called executive functions, which deal with executive control, planning, dealing with ambiguity, prioritizing, and multi-tasking. These skills are crucial to maintain independent living.

In this study, we examined whether playing a strategy-based video game can train those executive functions and improve them. We showed that playing a strategy-based videogame (Rise of Nations Gold Edition) could result in not only becoming a better videogame player but could also transfer to untrained executive functions. We saw a significant improvement in task switching, working memory, visual short-term memory, and mental rotation. And some, but more limited, benefits in inhibition and reasoning.

I can share a few details on the study: the average age of the participants was sixty-nine, and the experiment required around twenty-three hours of training time. We only included individuals who had played videogames zero hours per week for the previous two years.

That last criteria is interesting. We typically say that good "brain exercise" requires novelty, variety and challenge. So, if you take adults who are sixty-nine years old and have not played a videogame in two years, how do you know if the benefit comes from the particular videogame they played vs. just the value of dealing with a new and complex task?

That is a great question. The reality is that we do not know, since we had a "waiting list" control group. In the future perhaps we should compare different videogames or other mentally stimulating activities against each other and see what method is the most efficient. Perhaps the National Institutes on Health may be interested in funding such research.

In any case, your study reinforces an important point: older brains can, and do, learn new skills.

Yes. The rate of learning by older adults may be slower, and they may benefit from more explicit instruction and technology training; but, as a society, it is a massive waste of talent not to ensure that older adults remain active and productive.

Another recent study we conducted that is still under review is titled "Experience-Based Mitigation of Age-Related Performance Declines: Evidence from Air Traffic Control." It deals with the question: Can age itself be an obstacle for someone to perform as an air controller? And the answer is: age itself, within the age range that we studied, is not an obstacle. Our results suggest that, given substantial accumulated experience, older adults can be quite capable of performing at high levels of proficiency on fast-paced, demanding, real-world tasks like flying planes.

The field of computerized cognitive training has the potential to work in a variety of applications beyond "healthy aging". You are obviously familiar with Daniel Gopher's work training military pilots using Space Fortress. Is your lab doing something in the area of cognitive enhancement?

Yes, I have been involved in that area of work since the late 70s, when I helped design the protocols for Space Fortress. This program indeed provides a very interesting example of real-life transfer – pilots do seem to fly better as measured by real-life instruments.

Our lab is now embarking on a five years study for the U.S. Navy to explore ways to capitalize on emerging research about brain plasticity to enhance training and performance. MIT and my lab will analyze the best training procedures to increase the efficiency and efficacy of training of individual and team performance skills, particularly those skills requiring high levels of flexibility. The results from this study will be in the public domain, so I hope they will contribute to the maturity of the field at large.

MATURITY OF THE COGNITIVE FITNESS FIELD

That is an important point. What does the field of cognitive fitness at large need to mature and become more mainstream?

We need more research, but not just any kind of research. What we need is a kind of independent "seal of approval" based on independent clinical trials. Most published research of cognitive training interventions is sponsored and/or conducted by the companies themselves. We need independent, objective and clear standards of excellence.

The Department of Education maintains a "What Works Clearinghouse" to review existing evidence behind programs that make education-related claims. Perhaps we need a similar approach for programs making cognitive claims with adults. We also see a need for more solid and widely available cognitive assessments, to have better baselines and independent measures of cognitive abilities.

Good news there. The National Institute of Health is preparing an "NIH Toolbox" to provide valid, reliable instruments to researchers and clinicians, to solve the problem that exists today, namely, the lack of uniformity among the many measures used. This initiative was launched in 2006 and is a five years effort. So, we will need to wait to see results.

Interview with Dr. Elizabeth Zelinski – Healthy aging enhanced with computer-based programs.

BACKGROUND:

Dr. Elizabeth Zelinski of the Southern California Andrus Gerontology Center led the IMPACT (Improvement in Memory with Plasticity-based Adaptive Cognitive Training) study.

The IMPACT study, which is by far the largest high-quality study of its kind, was a prospective, randomized, controlled, and used a double blind trial. 524 healthy adults sixty-five or older were divided into two groups. One received an hour a day of brain training for eight to ten weeks, and the other spent the same amount of time watching educational DVDs. Funded by Posit Science corporation, the study was performed in multiple locations, including the Mayo Clinic, USCF, and San Francisco Veteran Affairs Medical Center.

HIGHLIGHTS:

- The aging brain has a harder time dealing with novelty but gets better at dealing with the familiar.
- There is not a general intelligence but many different cognitive abilities. This is why different programs need to be designed to train and improve each of them.

HOW COGNITIVE ABILITIES EVOLVE AS WE AGE

What insights did you gain from your Long Beach Longitudinal Study into how human cognitive abilities typically evolve as we age?

The first concept to understand is that different cognitive skills evolve over our lifespan in different ways. Some that rely on experience, such as vocabulary, actually improve as we age. Some tend to decline gradually, starting in our late twenties. This happens, for example, with processing speed (how long it takes us to process and respond to information), memory, and reasoning. We could summarize this phenomenon by saying that as we age we get better at dealing with the familiar, but worse at dealing with the new. We can always learn, but at a slower pace.

Is there a specific tipping or inflection point in this trend, any age when the rate of decline is more pronounced?

We do not have a clear answer to that. It depends a lot on the individual. In general it is a gradual, cumulative process, so that by age seventy we statistically see clear age declines. Which, for example, is a strong factor determining why older adults struggle to adapt to new technologies, but why trying to learn them provides needed mental stimulation. We know that genes only account for a portion of this decline. Much of it depends on our environment, lifestyle and actions.

Can you summarize what a healthy individual can do to slow down this process of decline, and help stay healthy and productive as long as possible?

One general recommendation is to do everything we can to prevent or delay disease processes, such as diabetes or high-blood pressure, that have a negative effect on our brains. For example, it is a tragedy in our society that we usually reduce our levels of physical exercise drastically after we leave school.

IMPACTS OF PHYSICAL VS. MENTAL EXERCISE

What are the relative virtues of physical vs. mental exercise?

This question leads to my second recommendation. Aerobic exercise has been shown to be a great contributor to overall cognitive health. But it has not shown any significant effect on improved memory. This is an important point to remember: there have been dozens of studies on the impact of physical exercise on cognition and they have found many impacts, but none in the area of memory. In contrast, directed cognitive training, or mental exercise, has been shown to improve specific cognitive abilities, including memory.

Now, there is no magic bullet. Both physical and mental exercise are important components. And I would add a third element: it is also important to maintain emotional connections. Not only with ourselves, to have self-confidence and self-esteem, but also with our family our friends.

IMPACT STUDY

What results of the IMPACT study surprised you the most?

Probably the most surprising outcome was a clear transfer of the training, which is critical so that the cognitive improvements have an impact on everyday life. The program we used, *Brain Fitness 2.0*, trains auditory processing. The people in the experimental group improved very significantly, which was not that surprising. What was very surprising was that there was also a clear benefit in auditory memory, which was not directly trained. In other words, we found that after using the program, people who were seventy-five years old performed auditory memory tasks as well as average sixty-five year olds, so we can say they reversed ten years of aging for that cognitive ability.

Another area where people in the experimental group showed significant improvement was in self-reported perception of their abilities in a variety of daily life tasks, such as remembering names and phone numbers, where they had left their keys, as well as communication abilities and feelings of self-confidence.

ENVISIONING A FUTURE WITH BRAIN GYMS

Those results, even if initial, are impressive and have very significant implications. Let us now speculate a bit about the future. We have said that different cognitive abilities evolve in different ways, and we have talked about just a few of them. We have discussed how physical exercise can be useful. And how directed cognitive training may help improve specific cognitive skills, like the Brain Fitness 2.0 program developed by Dr. Michael Merzenich. Other examples include working memory training, shown by Dr. Torkel Klingberg, and attentional control, by Dr. Daniel Gopher. In the future, will we have access to better assessments and tools to identify and train the cognitive abilities we need to work on the most, in the same way that we can go to a gym today and find the combination of machines that provide the most effective personalized workout?

The physical fitness analogy is a good one, in that cognitive enhancement requires engagement in a variety of activities. Those activities must be novel, adaptive and challenging. This is why computer-based programs can be helpful. Even at a more basic level, what matters is being engaged with life, continually exposed to stimulating activities, always trying to get out of our comfort zones, and doing our best at whatever we are doing.

A typical misconception about the brain is that there is only one general intelligence to care about. In reality, we have many different cognitive abilities, such as attention, memory, language, reasoning, and more, so it makes sense to have different programs designed to train and improve each of them. Before embarking on this study I was skeptical about what we would find. Now I believe that cognitive training is a very promising area that deserves more scientific and policy attention.

Chapter 3.

Mental Exercise vs. Mental Activity

HIGHLIGHTS

- Mental or brain exercise goes beyond mental activity. It is the structured use of cognitive exercises or techniques aimed at improving specific brain functions.
- Mental exercise (or brain training) can be delivered in a number of ways: meditation, cognitive therapy, cognitive training.
- Computerized brain training programs can help get a complete mental workout

In this chapter we focus on mental exercise – which we will call brain training, to clearly distinguish it from mental activity in general. First we try to define what brain training is. Then we highlight the different way you can get some brain training. Finally we focus on brain training software programs.

3.1. WHAT IS MENTAL EXERCISE OR "BRAIN TRAINING"?

In Chapter 2 we showed that brain maintenance includes balanced nutrition, stress management, physical exercise and brain exercise. We also reported that numerous studies have shown that intellectual activity in general is good for the brain and may help build up cognitive reserve.

The next question we need to clarify is, *How is brain training or brain exercise different from daily mental activities?* Let's take the example of physical activity. There is a clear difference between physical activity and physical exercise. Physical activity occurs whenever we move our body or engage in a leisure activity that involves moving our body (e.g., playing pool). Physical exercise (e.g. jogging) refers to the repeated and structured activity of particular parts of our bodies. While both physical activity and physical exercise may bring benefits, it is the latter that helps build capacity and muscles strength, contributing to staying fit as we age.

Similarly, brain "training", or brain "exercise", goes beyond mental activity. Mental activity takes place whenever one is awake, ranging from merely day dreaming to reading a book or learning a new language. **Mental exercise or brain training refers to the structured use of cognitive exercises or techniques. Its aim is to improve specific brain functions.**

Understanding the difference between mental activity and mental exercise is crucial. For instance, many people feel that they are doing the best for their brain after having completed their daily puzzle. However crossword puzzles challenge a relatively narrow range of cognitive skill and thus stimulate only a limited range of brain regions. A 1999 study showed that increased amount of experience in doing crossword puzzles does not modify the effect of age measured in tasks requiring vocabulary and reasoning (Hambrick et al.,1999). Crosswords puzzles generate mental activity but they do not constitute a brain training program!

This points out to the key word in brain training: variety. One needs a variety of challenging exercises in order to stimulate the whole brain. Recent recommendations made by a panel of experts reviewing a poll by the American Society on Aging (2006) stated: "A single activity, no matter how challenging, is not sufficient to sustain the kind of mental acuity that virtually everyone can achieve." Even if one's goal is to improve memory functions, other brain functions need stimulation to achieve that goal. For instance, attention and concentration are essential to good memorization.

Systematic brain training programs can be designed to lead to brain change in a more efficient way that random daily activities may. A combination of both may be ideal. Learning a complex skill such as learning the piano helps train and develop some parts of the brain. Well-designed training programs may help train and develop other parts.

Defined as the structured use of cognitive exercises or techniques aimed at improving specific brain functions, brain training includes a range of research-supported techniques or approaches, such as cognitive therapy and meditation, along with the most popular brain fitness software. This guide is focused on software programs but will also discuss other approaches.

3.2. DIFFERENT TYPES OF BRAIN TRAINING

Cognitive Therapy

Cognitive therapy (CT) was founded by Dr. Aaron Beck. It is based on the idea that the way people perceive their experience influences their behaviors and emotions. The therapist teaches the patient cognitive and behavioral skills to modify his or her dysfunctional thinking and actions.

CT aims at improving specific traits, behaviors, or cognitive skills, such as planning and flexibility, which are executive functions, depression, obsessive-compulsive disorders, and phobias. It has been shown effective in many studies and contexts such as depression, high levels of anxiety, insomnia. The interview with Lee Woodruff (Chapter 1) describes the spectacular recovery of her husband who suffered a severe traumatic brain injury in Iraq. CT was part of this recovery and was used to improve speech and language skills.

Recently, Dr. Aaron Beck's daughter, Dr. Judy Beck, has successfully used CT to help dieters acquire new skills in order to achieve their goals (see Dr. Beck's interview at the end of this Chapter). According to Dr. Beck, the main message of CT and its application in the diet world is that problems losing weight are not the dieter's fault. These problems reflect the lack of skills that can be acquired through training. What skills is Dr. Beck talking about? Mostly executive functions: the skills to plan in advance, to motivate oneself, to monitor one's behavior, etc.

Recent evidence supports the efficiency of CT. For instance, Stahre and Halstrom (2005) conducted a randomized controlled study testing the effect of CT on weight loss. Nearly all 65 patients completed the program and the short-term intervention (10-week, 30-hours) showed a significant long-term weight reduction, even larger (when compared to the 40 individuals in the control group) after 18 months than right after the 10-week program.

Neuroimaging has also been used to show the results of CT on the brain. Let's take the example of spider phobia. In 2003, Paquette and colleagues showed that before the cognitive therapy, the fear induced by viewing film clips depicting spiders was correlated with significant activation of specific brain areas, like the amygdala. After the intervention was completed (one three-hour group session per week, for four weeks), viewing the same spider films did not provoke activation of those areas. Dr. Judith Beck, explains that the adults in this study were able to "train their brains" which resulted in reducing the stress response triggered by spiders.

MEDITATION

You may be wondering what meditation has to do with brain training. In fact, meditation has been shown to improve specific cognitive functions such as attention. As such it can be considered as a brain training technique.

A number of studies have compared people who practice meditation to people who do not. The problem with these studies is that people in both groups can be very different. Thus the benefits observed in the group practicing meditation could be due to other things.

Recently, a more controlled study was conducted that showed a specific effect of meditation on attention, one of the main brain functions described in Chapter 1. In this study, Posner and his colleagues (2007) randomly assigned participants to either an Integrative Body-Mind Training (IBMT) or to a relaxation training. Both trainings lasted 5 days, 20mn per day. IBMT is a meditation technique developed in China in the 1990s. It stresses a balanced state of relaxation while focusing attention. Thought control is achieved with the help of a coach through posture, relaxation, body-mind harmony and balance. The results of this study showed that after training, participants in the IBMT training group showed more improvement in a task measuring executive attention than the control group. The IBMT training also helped reduced cortisol levels caused by mental stress.

Styles of meditation differ. Some technique use concentration meditation, mantra, mindfulness meditation, while others rely on body relaxation, breathing practice and mental imagery. It is not known so far what aspects of meditation or which techniques are the best to train one's brain. Scientists are researching what elements of meditation may help manage stress and improve memory. For instance, Dr. Andrew Newberg (whose interview can be found at the end of the present chapter) is currently conducting a study where 15 older adults with memory problems are practicing Kirtan Kriya meditation during 8 weeks. Preliminary results in terms of the impact on brain functions seem promising.

BIOFEEDBACK

Biofeedback hardware devices measure and graphically display various physiological variables such as skin conductivity and heart rate variability, so that users can learn to self-adjust. It has been used for decades in medicine. Recently, this technology has emerged in reasonably-priced applications for consumers who want to learn how to manage stress better.

Neurofeedback is a subset of biofeedback relying specifically on electrophysiological measures of brain activity. Using Electroencephalography (EEG) biofeedback to measure brain waves gives the user feedback on different "mental states" like alertness. Neurofeedback is still a tool mostly useful in research and highly specialized clinical contexts, not for mainstream healthcare and/or consumer applications, so we do not cover it in this guide.

Dr. Steenbarger, whose interview can be found at the end of the present chapter, recommends the use of relaxation coupled with biofeedback programs to improve trader's performance. These programs provide real-time visual feedback on a "trader's internal performance". You may be wondering how this may help a trader improve his or her performance? It is because of the close relationship between emotion and cognition. Emotion strongly affects cognition. Stress, as we mentioned earlier, can be very detrimental to performance. Thus, in jobs that are very emotional like trading, it is very important to learn how to self-regulate emotionally in order to improve one's cognitive performance According to Dr. Steenbarger, biofeedback programs can tell the traders whether they are in optimal conditions to learn and perform or whether they are becoming too stressed.

COMPUTER-BASED SOFTWARE

For many years, neuropsychologists have helped individuals suffering from traumatic brain injuries relearn how to talk, walk or make decisions, etc. Among other tools, cognitive exercises (including computer-assisted strategies) have been used to retrain abilities. However these tools are not available to the public and not everybody can afford a neuropsychologist or needs to see one. Things are changing as a variety of commercial programs is now making brain training available to the public. The challenge is to make informed decisions on which tools may be appropriate for specific needs and goals.

Since the launch of the original brain exercise hand-held computer game Brain Age (2005 in Japan, 2006 in the USA and Europe), Nintendo has proven that there is a large demand for mentally stimulating video games. These games can be seen as the next step in the chain after the traditional paper-based games such as crosswords and sudoku puzzles.

As of the end of January 2008, Nintendo has sold 17 million copies of brain exercise games worldwide since the launch of Brain Age in June 2005, with sales in the US trailing those in Japan and Europe. This success has attracted many imitation products from other gaming companies such as Sega (which released their own brain game in Japan before Nintendo, without comparable success), Majesco and Ubisoft.

3.3. BRAIN TRAINING SOFTWARE: AN EMERGING FIELD

Structured sets of brain exercises designed to train specific brain areas and functions have been used by the military and by clinical neuropsychologists for a long time. What is happening now is that this approach is being repackaged and commercialized for new and wider audiences.

We define "brain training software" as fully-automated applications designed to assess and enhance cognitive abilities. Adaptive software-based programs present the user with various tools to exercise different brain structures and cognitive skills by continually responding to performance and increasing difficulty level incrementally. From now on we will focus on such programs.

These software products can be delivered either online (such as www. lumosity.com), via software (such as Posit Science Brain Fitness Program Classic), or can be used on devices (such as Nintendo's Brain Age). The products can be either sold directly to consumers or via authorized clinicians (such as NovaVision and Cogmed).

Over the past few years, a few software companies have achieved commercial success in selling brain exercises to consumer and institutional buyers. Several companies have commercialized programs designed to alleviate specific conditions, such as attention deficit disorder, dyslexia or stroke-related vision problems. Others have launched products with broader healthy aging goals in mind.

Brain training software-based programs can complement and enhance other common daily activities. They are probably the best-suited format to deliver a calibrated mix of novelty and variety at constantly evolving levels of difficulty that ensure constant challenge.

3.4. DO BRAIN TRAINING SOFTWARE PROGRAMS REALLY "WORK"?

To determine if something works we first need to define what we mean by "work". A machine to train abdominal muscles probably won't "work" if what we measure is blood pressure. In the same way, a program training auditory processing speed may not work if visual functions are measured (see Chapter 1 for a better understanding of cognitive abilities). This is why to determine whether a brain training software "works" it is crucial to (a) understand the claims made by the developer as to what abilities are trained, (b) find well conducted studies showing that these abilities are indeed trained by the program and (c) decide whether that training is relevant to one's needs and objectives.

Another important aspect when evaluating whether a brain training program "works" is to look at the extend to which the training effects transfer to untrained tasks. It is well established that practice usually triggers improvement in the practiced tasks. So the first requirement for a well working brain training program is to show that people who use the program get better at the tasks trained. The second and more important requirement is to show that this improvement transfers to other, untrained, tasks, mostly tasks performed during everyday life. This would show that the cognitive abilities targeted by the program were indeed trained. If I use a training program to train my ability to concentrate (attention skills) I will probably get better at the tasks included in the program if I practice long enough, but will I see any benefits when I do other tasks, at work for instance?

Teams of neuroscientists and psychologists from around the world have partnered with software and game developers to bring targeted brain fitness products to market with more solid clinical validation. These teams have published results using the gold standard of randomized controlled trials, supported by neuroimaging. As a result, they have been able to claim quantifiable short-term and long-term improvements to specific cognitive skills if used according to a specific regimen over a specified length of time.

Much of the hope and media coverage of the brain fitness market in 2007 can be traced to the publication of the results of the five years ACTIVE study conducted by Willis and her colleagues (2001, 2006). This study was one of the first randomized controlled, scientifically sound studies ever published in the area of brain training. Participants in this groundbreaking study were 73.6 years old on average. They were exposed to different forms of mental training: reasoning, memory and speed training. Strategies and practice were provided during training. The training of processing speed was computer-based. Participants showed an improvement in the skills trained and retained a significant percentage of this improvement when tested five years later. Interestingly, the group who received the training in processing speed showed the most pronounced short-term and long-term improvements.

Since the publication of the ACTIVE study, a growing number of randomized controlled studies are showing how well directed training software may produce cognitive and other improvements to daily life.

For instance, in 1994, Dr. Daniel Gopher and his colleagues used Space Fortress, a complex computer game precursor to IntelliGym, to train flight cadets. Participants received 10h of training. Results showed that compared to a no-training group, flight cadets who were trained showed a 30% improvement in their flight performance. This supports the idea that the benefit gained through practicing a computer game can transfer to a task involving similar cognitive abilities (flight performance here).

Cogmed is a computerized program aimed at improving working memory (WM). WM is the memory system that allows one to hold information briefly in mind for the purpose of the task at hand. In 2005, Dr. Torkel Klingberg and his colleagues conducted a randomized, controlled, study to test whether the use of Cogmed could help improve the WM performance of children with attention-deficit/hyperactivity disorder (ADHD). The training period was at least 20 days. Results showed that training WM using Cogmed increased the performance of the children in untrained tasks measuring WM as well as in tasks measuring response inhibition and complex reasoning. The benefits were still present when the children were tested again 3 month after the training.

Dr. Arthur Kramer, whose interview you can find at the end of Chapter 2, just published the results of a study testing the benefits induced by playing a strategy-based videogame (Rise of Nations Gold Edition). Results of this study showed that trained participants (age 69 on average) not only got better at playing the game but also showed transfer of benefits to untrained tasks that engaged the same abilities (working memory, task switching, etc.) as the game.

In 2003, Dr. John Gabrieli and his colleagues used Fast Forword, a computerized program designed to train auditory processing with 20 children with dyslexia. Functional Magnetic Resonance Imaging (fMRI) was performed on the children during phonological processing before and after the training. Behaviorally, the training improved oral language and reading performance. Physiologically, children with dyslexia showed increased activity in multiple brain areas correlated with improvement in oral language ability. These results suggest that the training improved the targeted brain functions. Although the number of participants in this study was small, the results were replicated in a further study published in 2007.

Posit Science Classic is another computerized program, designed to train auditory processing. One controlled, randomized, study published in 2006 by Dr. Michael Merzenich and his colleagues showed that adults age 60 and over trained using Posit Science program improved in auditory tasks. More importantly the improvement generalized to an untrained memory task. The memory benefits were still present 3 months after the training. The same computerized program is ongoing further testing in the IMPACT study conducted by Dr. Elizabeth Zelinski (see her interview at the end of Chapter 2). The initial results of this study were presented at the Gerontology Society of America in 2007. They showed significant gains in auditory processing and auditory memory "equivalent to ten years of aging for that skill" in over 500 adults with a median age of seventy-five.

In sum, these studies show quantifiable improvements to specific cognitive skills if the tested brain training software is used according to a specific regimen over a specified length of time. In some studies, transfer of benefit to untrained tasks has also been observed.

However, it is still too early to tell whether or not these products will result in measurable long-term health benefits, such as better overall brain health, or lower incidence of Alzheimer's symptoms. One of the reasons for this, to be fair, is the fact that most of the commercially available products have not been on the market long enough to examine any longer term effects.

Note that not all companies are running randomized, controlled, studies to show that their product has a specific impact on brain functions. These companies, such as Nintendo, base their more limited claims on general research that shows how mental stimulation can lower the probability of developing Alzheimer's and other dementias' symptoms, via the cognitive reserve theory. We can view these untested programs as a new, high-tech, generation of crossword puzzles, that may be useful but that cannot make specific brain benefit claims beyond the general "use it or lose it."

3.5. FLOOD OF BRAIN TRAINING SOFTWARE WITHOUT TAXONOMY

Brain training is now a household expression for many families, courtesy of Nintendo. What is less visible than Nintendo's success is the growing number of science-based companies that aim to train specific cognitive skills. Posit Science has been getting increasing levels of attention, including a PBS Special. Yet, consumers struggle to understand the potential value of this auditory processing intervention as opposed to doing one more crossword puzzle, or buying a Nintendo game.

A new generation of products include those by Posit Science (Brain Fitness Program Classic and Insight), CogniFit (MindFit), Lumos Labs (Lumosity.com), Scientific Brain Training (Happy-Neuron.com), and others, that add options to earlier attempts, such as those by MyBrainTrainer and BrainBuilder.

There needs to be a common taxonomy, perhaps similar to how food labels clarify the ingredients, to educate consumers on what cognitive benefits those products are aimed at and with what specific evidence.

We believe that over time consumers and healthcare professionals will become more sophisticated in their shopping habits. They will evaluate programs using criteria similar to the SharpBrains checklist presented in Chapter 4. They will also learn to make sure that the product they are considering has been validated via solid randomized, controlled, studies. Importantly, brain training users will also learn how to determine what cognitive enhancements they need and which program may help deliver those.

3.6. INTERVIEWS

- Dr. Judith Beck: The link between brain training and weight loss.
- Dr. Andrew Newberg: The value of meditation.
- Dr. Brett Steenbarger: Achieving peak performance in high-pressure professions.
- Dr. Martin Buschkuehl: Can intelligence be trained?
- Dr. Arthur Lavin: Working memory training at a pediatrician office.

Interview with Dr. Judith Beck – The link between brain training and weight loss.

BACKGROUND:

Dr. Judith Beck is the Director of the Beck Institute for Cognitive Therapy and Research and a Clinical Associate Professor of psychology at the University of Pennsylvania. Dr. Beck is the author of *Cognitive Therapy: Basics and Beyond*. Her most recent book is *The Beck Diet Solution: Train Your Brain to Think Like a Thin Person*.

HIGHLIGHTS:

- Cognitive therapy teaches cognitive and behavioral skills to modify dysfunctional thinking and actions.
- Cognitive therapy can help dieters acquire new skills to achieve their goal.

LINKING COGNITIVE THERAPY TO WEIGHT LOSS

What is cognitive therapy?

Cognitive therapy, as developed by my father Aaron Beck, is a comprehensive system of psychotherapy, based on the idea that the way people perceive their experience influences their emotional, behavioral, and physiological responses. Part of what cognitive therapists do is to help people solve the problems they are facing today. We also teach cognitive and behavioral skills to modify dysfunctional thinking and actions.

What motivated you to bring cognitive therapy techniques to the weight-loss field by writing "The Beck Diet Solution"?

Since the beginning, I have primarily treated psychiatric outpatients with a variety of diagnoses, especially depression and anxiety. Some patients expressed weight loss as a secondary goal in treatment. I found that many of the same cognitive and behavioral techniques that helped them overcome their other problems could also help them lose weight – and keep it off.

I became particularly interested in the problem of being overweight and was able to identify specific mindsets or cognitions about food, eating, hunger, craving, perfectionism, helplessness, self-image, unfairness, deprivation, and others that needed to be targeted to help them reach their goal.

What research results back your finding that those techniques help people lose weight and keep it off?

Probably the best study published so far is the randomized controlled study by Karolinska Institute's Stahre and Hallstrom (2005). The results were striking: nearly all sixty-five patients completed the program and this short-term intervention (ten weeks, thirty hours/week) showed significant long-term weight reduction. The results were even larger, when compared to the forty individuals in the control group after eighteen months than right after the ten weeks program.

That sounds impressive. Can you explain what makes this approach so effective?

My book does not offer a diet. But, it does provide tools to develop the mindset that is required for sustainable success, for modifying sabotaging thoughts and behaviors that typically follow people's initial good intentions. I help dieters acquire new skills.

So, could we say that your book is complementary to all other diet books?

Exactly – it helps readers set and reach their long-term goals, assuming that their diet is healthy, nutritious, and well balanced.

The main message of cognitive therapy overall, and its application in the diet world, is straightforward: problems losing weight are not a dieter's fault. Problems simply reflect lack of skills that can be acquired and mastered through practice. Dieters who read the book or workbook learn a new cognitive or behavioral skill every day for six weeks. They may practice some skills just once and incorporate others for their lifetime.

HOW TO USE COGNITIVE SKILLS TO OVERCOME CRAVINGS

What are the cognitive and emotional skills and habits that dieters need to train?

The key ones are:

- *How to motivate oneself.* The first task that dieters do is to write a list of the 15 of 20 reasons they want to lose weight and read that list to themselves every single day.
- *Planning in advance and self-monitoring behavior.* A typical reason for diet failure is a strong preference for spontaneity. I ask people to prepare a plan and then I teach them the skills to stick to it.
- *Overcome sabotaging thoughts.* Dieters have hundreds and hundreds of thoughts that lead them to engage in unhelpful eating behavior. I have dieters read cards that remind them of key points, such as: it is not worth the few moments of pleasure they will get from eating something they had not planned and that they will feel badly afterwards; that they cannot eat whatever they want, whenever they want, in whatever quantity they want, and still be thinner; that the scale is not supposed to go down every single day; and that they deserve credit for each helpful eating behavior they engage in, to name just a few.
- *Tolerate hunger and craving.* Overweight people often confuse the two. You experience hunger when your stomach feels empty. Craving is an urge to eat, usually experienced in the mouth or throat, even if your stomach is full.

When do people typically experience cravings?

Triggers can be environmental (seeing or smelling food), biological (hormonal changes), social (being with others who are eating), mental (thinking about or imagining tempting food), or emotional (wanting to soothe yourself when you're upset). The trigger itself is less important than what you do about it. Dieters need to learn exactly what to say to themselves and what to do when they have cravings so they can wait until their next planned meal or snack.

How can people learn that they do not have to eat in response to hunger or craving?

I ask dieters, once they get medical clearance, to skip lunch one day and not eat between breakfast and dinner. Just doing this exercise once proves to dieters that hunger is never an emergency; that it is tolerable; that it does not keep getting worse, but instead, comes and goes; and that they do not need to "fix" their usually mild discomfort by eating.

This exercise helps dieters lose a fear of hunger. It also teaches alternative actions to help refocus attention. Feel hungry? Well, try calling a friend, taking a walk, playing a computer game, doing some email, reading a diet book, surfing the net, brushing your teeth, or doing a puzzle.

My ultimate goal is to train dieters to resist temptations by firmly saying "Eating now is not my choice," to themselves, and then naturally turning their attention back to what they had been doing or engaging in whatever activity comes next.

You said earlier that some cravings follow an emotional reaction to stressful situations. Can you elaborate on that, and explain how cognitive techniques help?

In the short term, the most effective way is to identify the problem and try to solve it. If there is nothing you can do at the moment, call a friend, do deep breathing or relaxation exercises, take a walk to clear your mind, or distract yourself in another way. Read a card that reminds you that you will certainly not be able to lose weight or keep it off if you constantly turn to food to comfort yourself when you are upset. People without weight problems generally do not turn to food when they are upset. Dieters can learn to do other things, too.

And in the long term, I encourage people to examine and change their underlying beliefs and internal rules. Many people, for example, want to do everything (and expect others to do everything) in a perfect way one hundred percent of the time. That is simply impossible. This kind of thinking leads to stress.

COGNITIVE THERAPY'S IMPACT ON THE BRAIN

The title of your book includes a "train your brain" promise. Can you tell us a bit about the growing literature that analyzes the neurobiological impact of cognitive therapy?

Yes, that is a very exciting area. For years, we could only measure the impact of cognitive therapy based on psychological assessments. Today, thanks to fMRI and other neuroimaging techniques, we are starting to understand the impact our actions can have on specific parts of the brain.

For example, take spider-phobia. In a 2003 paper scientists (Paquette and colleagues) observed how, prior to the therapy, the fear induced by viewing film clips depicting spiders was correlated with significant activation of specific brain areas, like the amygdala. After the intervention was complete (one three-hour group session per week for four weeks), viewing the same spider films did not provoke activation of those areas. Those adults were able to train their brains and reduce the brain response that typically triggers automatic stress responses.

That is exactly what we find most exciting about this emerging field of neuroplasticity: the awareness that we can improve our lives by refining or "training" our brains, and the growing research behind a number of tools such as cognitive therapy.

Interview with Dr. Andrew Newberg – The value of meditation.

BACKGROUND:

Dr. Andrew Newberg is an Associate Professor in the Department of Radiology and Psychiatry and Adjunct Assistant Professor in the Department of Religious Studies at the University of Pennsylvania. He has published a variety of neuroimaging studies related to aging and dementia. He has also researched the neurophysiological correlates of meditation, prayer, and how brain function is associated with mystical and religious experiences.

HIGHLIGHTS:

- Scientists are researching what elements of meditation may help manage stress and improve memory.
- Meditation requires practice and dedication: ongoing research focuses on techniques that would be easier to teach and practice.

MEDITATION MAY HELP MANAGE STRESS AND IMPROVE MEMORY

Dr. Newberg, thank you for being with us today. Can you please explain the source of your interests at the intersection of brain research and spirituality?

Since I was a kid, I had a keen interest in spiritual practice. I always wondered how spirituality and religion affect us, and over time I came to appreciate how science can help us explore and understand the world around us, including why we humans care about spiritual practices. This, of course, led me to be particularly interested in brain research.

During medical school I was particularly attracted by the problem of consciousness. I was fortunate to meet researcher Dr. Eugene D'Aquili in the early 1990s, who had been doing much research on religious practices' effect on the brain since the 1970s. Through him I came to see that brain imaging can provide a fascinating window into the brain.

Can we define religion and spirituality -which sound to me as very different brain processes-, and why learning about them may be helpful from a purely secular, scientific point of view?

Good point, definitions matter, since different people may be searching for God in different ways. I view being religious as participating in organized rituals and shared beliefs, such as going to church. Being spiritual, on the other hand, is more of an individual practice, whether we call it meditation, or relaxation, or prayer, aimed at expanding the self, developing a sense of oneness with the universe.

What is happening is that specific practices that have traditionally been associated with religious and spiritual contexts may also be very useful from a mainstream, secular, health point of view, beyond those contexts. Scientists are researching, for example, what elements of meditation may help manage stress and improve memory. How breathing and meditation techniques can contribute to health and wellness. For example, my lab is now conducting a study where 15 older adults with memory problems are practicing Kirtan Kriya meditation during 8 weeks, and we have found very promising preliminary outcomes in terms of the impact on brain function. This work is being funded by the Alzheimer's Research and Prevention Foundation, but we have submitted a grant request to the National Institute of Health as well.

Can you give an overview of the benefits of meditation, including Richard Davidson's studies on mindfulness meditation?

There are many types of meditation - and we each are researching different practices - which of course share some common elements, but are different in nature. Dr. Davidson has access to the Dalai Lama and many Buddhist practitioners, so much of his research centers on mindfulness meditation. We have easier access to Franciscan monks and to practitioners of Kirtan Kriya meditation.

At its core, meditation is an active process that requires alertness and attention, which explains why we often find increased brain activity in frontal lobes during practice. Usually you need to focus on something - a mantra, a visual or verbal prompt- while you monitor breathing.

A variety of studies have already shown the stress management benefits of meditation, resulting in what is often called Mindfulness Based Stress Reduction. What we are researching now is what are the cognitive - attention, memory- benefits? It is clear that memory depends on attention and the ability to screen out distractions - so we want to measure the effect of meditation on the brain, both structurally and functionally.

To measure the brain activation patterns we have been using SPECT imaging, which involves injecting small amounts of radioactive tracers in volunteers, and helps us get a better view of what happens during practice (fMRI is much more noisy).

To measure functional benefits we use the typical batteries of neuropsychology testing.

MEDITATION IN EVERYDAY LIFE

If there is a growing body of evidence behind the health and cognitive benefits of meditation - what is preventing a more widespread adoption of the practice, perhaps in ways similar to yoga, which is now pretty much a mainstream activity?

Well, the reality is that meditation requires practice and dedication. It is not an easy fix. And some of the best-researched meditation techniques, such as mindfulness meditation, are very intensive. You need a trained facilitator. You need to stick to the practice.

In fact, that's why our ongoing research focused on a much easier to teach and practice technique. We want to see if people can practice on their own, at home, a few minutes a day for a few weeks.

The other problem is that this is not a standardized practice, so there is a lot of confusion: many different meditation techniques, with different sets of priorities and styles.

My advice for interested people would be to look for something simple, easy to try first, ensuring the practice is compatible with one's beliefs and goals. You need to match practice with need: understand the specific goals you have in mind, your schedule and lifestyle, and find something practical. Otherwise, you will not stick to it (similar to people who never show up at the health club despite paying fees).

New York Times columnist David Brooks recently wrote two very thought-provoking articles, one on the Cognitive Age we are living in, another on the Neural Buddhists, where he quotes your work. What is the big picture, the main implications for society from your research?

I believe Philosophy complements Science, and all of us human beings would benefit from spiritual practices to achieve higher state of being, develop compassion, increase awareness, in ways compatible with any religious or secular beliefs. This is the main theme of my upcoming book, *How God Changes Brain* (to be published on March 2009): how we develop a shared knowledge of our common biology, and celebrate the differences which are based on our specific contexts. We are spiritual and social beings.

From an education point of view, I believe schools will need to recognize that rote learning is not enough, and add to the mix practices to improve cognition, and manage stress and relationships.

That spiritual angle may prove controversial in a number of scientific quarters. What would you, for example, say to biologist Richard Dawkins?

I'd tell him that we all view the world through the lens of our brains, reflecting our cultural, social, and personal background. His view is based on his lens. Same as mine. All of us have a belief system. His is not particularly more accurate than everybody else's.

We shouldn't throw out the baby with bathwater. I don't think religion is a black & white matter: yes, fundamentalism is a problem, as is rejecting data and ignoring scientific findings. But there are also good elements: the motivation to care about human beings, to develop compassion, to perfect ourselves and our world.

Interview with Dr. Brett Steenbarger – Achieving peak performance in high-pressure professions.

BACKGROUND:

The applications of cognitive neuroscience to trading and finance are central to Dr. Brett Steenbarger's research. Dr. Steenbarter wears many hats, including Associate Professor of Psychiatry and Behavioral Sciences at SUNY Upstate Medical University, active trader of over 30 years, former Director of Trader Development for Kingstree Trading, LLC, and author of *The Psychology of Trading: Tools and Techniques for Minding the Markets* and the recent *Enhancing Trader Performance: Proven Strategies From the Cutting Edge of Trading Psychology*. He writes feature columns for the *Trading Markets website* and several trading publications, including *Stocks Futures and Options*.

HIGHLIGHTS:

- Traders would benefit from following the example of elite performers and have many tools at their disposal – including books, simulation programs, biofeedback programs for emotional management, and coaches.
- Many people who do not end up performing at a high level are not motivated to follow the same level of intensive and systematic training as elite performers.

WHAT TRADERS AND OTHER PROFESSIONALS CAN LEARN FROM ELITE PERFORMERS

Give us some context on your interest in trading performance and how it led you to your new book.

My main interest is how to enhance cognitive and emotional development among traders to help them become more successful. My first book, *The Psychology of Trading*, focused on emotional and stress management, and tried to help traders – both professionals and amateurs – overcome the emotional disruptions of trading. My new book, *Enhancing Trader Performance*, helps traders develop their own training programs or, we may even call them, "brain gyms," to build their skills, strengthen their mental capacities, and improve their performance.

What is the premise of your new book, Enhancing Trader Performance?

The premise is that elite performers in highly competitive fields share common traits. This includes people in such fields as athletics, performing arts, chess, the military, and medicine. I review the research regarding what makes people successful in those fields, find the common factors behind their success, and then apply the findings to traders.

What are those common factors for top performers? And what differentiates elite performers from the rest?

The elite performers are most distinguished by the structure of their learning process. From a relatively early age, they are engaged in an intensive learning process that builds upon their natural talents. They find a niche – a field that makes use of their talents – and become absorbed by a deliberative and systematic learning process that provides them with continuous feedback about their performance.

The recipe for success seems to be talent, skill, hard work, and opportunity. In contrast, many people who do not end up performing at a high level are driven mostly by practical reasons to enter a given field and are not motivated to follow the same level of intensive and systematic training as the elite performers.

What type of training and practice will help traders function at peak performance levels?

Traders typically devote little time to practice and a structured learning process. I want to encourage them to see that "learning on the job" is not a substitute for breaking down skills into components, drilling these, receiving feedback about performance, and making continuous modifications and improvements.

In every field, elite performers devote more time to practice than to the actual performance. To perform at the highest level, you need to protect and optimize practice and learning time. The average trader does not do that, and the result is that many traders lose their trading capital within seven months of trading. To develop themselves, I suggest traders structure their learning processes.

There are several elements to this development:
- *Simulation and Biofeedback Tools*: There are very good simulations out there that can help traders become more sensitive to patterns in the market and internalize these. The ability to play and replay market days provides traders with enhanced screen time to accelerate and deepen learning. Another set of tools includes biofeedback programs that help traders manage their emotions. Biofeedback is especially helpful in reducing emotional arousal that can disrupt executive functions such as judgment, planning, analyzing, and reasoning.
- *Reflection and Regular Feedback:* Traders who utilize programs to provide them with metrics on their trading performance – analyses of their winning and losing trades – have considerable data at their disposal. The

patterns revealed by these metrics help traders figure out both strengths and weaknesses. Many times, building on successes is more important than trying to change weaknesses. Constant feedback on trading results shows traders what they do best – and help them do more of it.

- *Role of Mentors and Coaches:* In many performance fields, such as music and tennis, coaches help students break down their performance into component skills and then systematically work on these individually and in combination. The mentor is someone who can structure the learning process for the developing performer and help them move along the path from being a novice to being competent to being expert. Both are useful for traders.

Interesting analogy. Who would be a good "trader coach" and where does one find one?

Ideally, you need an experienced and successful trader who is familiar with the kind of trading that you will be doing. The book contains an appendix with different resources that can help traders find educational and mentoring resources. For emotional development, traders can also coach themselves with practical cognitive and behavioral techniques and build new, positive ways of thinking and behaving. The last two chapters of the book provide readers with self-help manuals for utilizing these techniques.

What are the key components of top performance in trading, and what skills traders can develop?

First, we must differentiate between short-term and long-term traders. For short-term traders, the priority is the ability to process large amounts of information and to quickly see patterns that will lead to effective decision making. They need speed, and good working memory. For long-term traders, analytical skills are paramount.

For both, I would add, knowing how to deal with "the emotional factor" is very important. Many traders get very frustrated when their bets do not go the way they expected, and become paralyzed or make non-logical decisions. Others may lose concentration and focus when they get fatigued, and make impulsive decisions. But I would stress that there is more to trading success than controlling emotions. It takes talent, skill, and a constant learning process.

I would also emphasize that, yes, we can train and get better at many things, but it is equally important to ensure an optimal fit between our trading talents and interests: the markets we trade and the ways we trade them. There has to be a fit between what we're good at and the opportunities afforded by a particular market and trading style.

How applicable are these findings to professionals in other fields?

People who aspire to be top performers in any field must build on what comes naturally to them, in order to be truly motivated and absorb constant learning. They will need to structure programs to develop their skills and work these programs diligently. Because elite performers do what comes naturally, they become absorbed in the development of their skills. If you have to motivate yourself to work at something, it is probably not your calling.

BRAIN TRAINING PROGRAMS: NOW AND IN THE FUTURE

What training programs are available today and which ones do you foresee will be available in the future?

First, I find that Dr. Elkhonon Goldberg's metaphor of a gymnasium for the brain is very appealing. We will be seeing more and more tools for cognitive and brain fitness. Dr. Goldberg cites considerable research that indicates we can improve the functioning of our frontal cortex - home of our executive functions such as reasoning, planning, judgment, analysis, and problem-solving – through structured exercises, much as we can build muscles in the gym.

Today, traders have very realistic simulation programs that can help them identify market patterns and improve decision making. True, as Professor Gopher said in your interview with him, what matters is the cognitive fidelity of those simulations, and how they will help traders see new, non-historical, patterns. But, at the very least, existing simulation packages help traders learn very quickly how to identify a wealth of recurring patterns in markets.

Finally, I work with many traders on their emotional reactions – especially new traders. Behavioral techniques can be very helpful to develop calmer, open minds and good attitudes. In a blog post, I stress the need to keep an open mind and avoid missing unexpected "gorillas" in the market. We need to be aware of and manage the narrowing of our attention that usually follows hyper-focus. For the many people out there who become angry and frustrated after trading losses, I recommend exercises such as deep breathing and visual imagery, which, after a period of practice, can be applied very quickly to our work when we need it. These techniques can be reinforced by the use of biofeedback programs that provide real-time visual feedback on a trader's "internal performance." The biofeedback programs reveal whether traders are in the zone of optimal learning and performance or are becoming too stressed, anxious, and impulsive.

It is important to understand the role of emotions: they are not "bad". They are very useful signals. It is, however, important to become aware of them to avoid being engulfed by them, and to learn how to manage them.

Interview with Martin Buschkuehl – Can intelligence be trained?

BACKGROUND:

Dr. Martin Buschkuehl is a researcher at the University of Michigan's Cognitive Neuroimaging Lab. He is one of the primary researchers involved in the cognitive training study, called "Improving Fluid Intelligence with Training on Working Memory," that has received a great deal of media attention. The study was published in April 2008 in the Proceedings of the National Academy of Sciences.

HIGHLIGHTS:

- Fluid intelligence, which may be defined as the ability to deal with new problems, can be improved with training on a working memory task.
- Transfer of working memory training benefits can be observed from one task to another.

CAN INTELLIGENCE BE IMPROVED?

Can you first provide us with some context on your research?

My collaborator Susanne Jaeggi and I started our training work four years ago in the Lab of Professor Walter Perrig at the University of Bern in Switzerland. Now we are both Post Docs in Professor John Joindes' Lab at the University of Michigan. The publication in the Proceedings of the National Academy of Science is the first time our training work has been published in a peer-reviewed journal.

Could you please explain the training involved in this particular study?

We recruited 70 students around 26 years old and set half of them on a challenging computer-based cognitive training regimen, based on the so-called "n-back task." This is a very complex working memory task that involves the simultaneous presentation of visual and auditory stimuli. ("Working Memory" is the ability to hold several units of information in the mind and to manipulate them in real time.) The experimental group watched a series of screens on their computers, where a blue square appeared in various positions on a black background. Each screen appeared for half a second, with a 2.5 second gap before the next one appeared. While this happened, the trainees also heard a series of letters that were read out at the same rate.

At first, students had to say if either the screen or the letter matched those that popped up two cycles ago. The number of cycles increased or decreased depending on how well the students performed the task. The students sat through about twenty-five minutes of training per day for either eight, twelve, seventeen, or nineteen days. They were tested on their fluid intelligence before and after the regimen using the Bochumer-Matrizen Test. The Bochumer-Matrizen Test is a problem-solving task based on the same principle as the very well known Raven's Advanced Progressive Matrices. However, it is more difficult and therefore especially suited for academic samples.

What were the results?

Participants in the experimental group did significantly better on the fluid intelligence test, which was not directly trained, than the participants in the control group. "Fluid intelligence" can be described as the ability to deal with new challenges and new problems that we encounter for the first time. Those in the control group had not gone through any training. The control group did improve slightly, but the real "trainees" outperformed them. Furthermore, we found that the improvement was dose-dependent: the more they trained, the larger the gain on fluid intelligence.

What are the particular aspects of this study that surprised you the most?

First, the clear transfer into fluid intelligence that many researchers and psychologists assume is fixed.

Second, I was surprised to see that the more training, the better the outcome. The improvements did not seem to peak early.

Third, that all trained groups improved, no matter their respective starting points. In fact, students with the lowest fluid intelligence seemed to improve the most. But that was not the main focus of our study, so we cannot say much more about it.

BENEFITS OF USING COMPUTERIZED BRAIN TRAINING PROGRAMS

A common question we get about brain training software is, How are computerized programs like the one you used fundamentally different from, say, simply doing many crossword puzzles?

In terms of why our program worked, I could say that the program has some inherent properties that are, at least in this combination, unique to our training approach.

Our program is:

– Fully adaptive in real-time: The person using the program is truly pushed to his or her peak level all the time, thereby "stretching" the targeted ability.
– Complex: We present a very complex task, mixing different forms of stimuli (auditory and visual) under time pressure.

– Designed for transferability: The tasks are designed in a way that does not allow for the development of task-specific "strategies" to beat the game. If one truly expands working memory capacity, this helps to ensure the transfer to non-trained tasks.

This is very different from enhancing task-specific capacities, such as memorizing lists of 100 numbers, which have been shown not to necessarily transfer to related domains.

Can you give an example of the lack of transferability of other training methods?

In Ericsson's (1998) classic paper, people who could memorize one hundred numbers using a variety of mnemonic techniques could not get even close to one hundred letters. Remembering numbers did not translate into remembering other things, so it was not a general memory capacity that had been improved.

How did participants describe the experience, and their benefits?

Many liked the training. They saw the challenge, and tried hard to push themselves through the training to see how far they could go.

We did not analyze how the fluid intelligence gains transferred into real life. But from an anecdotal point of view, many participants have shared stories of how they perceive a major benefit. Now they can follow lectures more easily, understand math better etc.

DEBATING PHYSICAL VS. MENTAL EXERCISE

There is a degree of artificial controversy these days in the media and the scientific community on the respective benefits of physical or mental exercise. What are your thoughts on the value of the different types of exercise?

We obviously need both. Physical exercise keeps the body in a good shape but especially in older people also leads to cognitive benefits. Mental exercise, like the one we used, can enhance important abilities and is most likely the most efficient way to improve a specific cognitive process but also generalizes to a broader range of skills, as we showed.

Research will need to be done to help clarify who needs what type of exercise more. Some people may get enough mental exercise through very complex jobs and what they need is physical exercise. For others, it may be the opposite.

NEXT STEPS

What are your plans now?

First, to conduct follow-up neuroimaging studies to analyze the neural basis of the improvement and second, to try to measure the benefits in real life. Our main hope is to be able to investigate and develop applications for people who need the improvement the most: children with development problems, stroke/ Traumatic Brain Injury rehabilitation, and older adults.

Also, let me note that there is a cross-platform application available to train the dual n-back task and several other training tasks that we developed for other studies. Although the application is available in English, the Manual and the BrainTwister Website are not at the moment. We are about to release an English version, but unfortunately I cannot give you a release date right now. If the training program is used for research (i.e. a training study), it is provided free of charge.

Interview with Dr. Arthur Lavin – Working memory training at a pediatrician office.

BACKGROUND:

Dr. Arthur Lavin is an Associate Clinical Professor of Pediatrics at Case Western School of Medicine. He is also a pediatrician in private practice and one of the first providers of Cogmed Working Memory Training in the US. Dr. Lavin has a long standing interest in technology – as evidenced by Microsoft's recognition of his paperless office – and in brain research and applications. He trained with esteemed Dr. Mel Levine who wrote *All Kinds of Minds*.

Dr. Lavin opens the way for new interventions and public policies incorporating an understanding of what "education" and "learning" is and how to "educate" millions of young minds and equip them for life success.

HIGHLIGHTS:

- Schools today are not yet in a position to effectively help kids with cognitive issues deal with increasing cognitive demands.
- Working memory can be trained.

COGNITIVE FITNESS AND SCHOOLS

It is not very common for a pediatrician to have such an active interest in brain research and cognitive fitness. Can you explain the source of your interest?

Throughout my life I have been fascinated by how the mind works. Both from the research point of view and the practical one: how can scientists' increasing knowledge improve kids' lives? We now live in a truly exciting era in which solid scientific progress in neuroscience is at last creating opportunities to improve people's actual cognitive function. The progress Cogmed has achieved in creating a program that can make great differences in the lives of children with attention deficits is one of the most exciting recent developments.

My colleague Susan Glaser and I recently published two books: *Who's Boss: Moving Families from Conflict to Collaboration* and *Baby and Toddler Sleep Solutions for Dummies*. So, I see myself not only as a pediatrician but also as an educator. I see parents in real need of guidance and support.

Parents are usually both very skeptical, since they have been promised too many things too many times by "experts", and open-minded to ideas with good foundations. Many professionals have only the skeptical frame of mind, since they were educated when scientists still believed the brain was pretty rigid and "un-trainable". We need much more brain science based professional development.

BARRIERS TO INCORPORATING BRAIN GYMS IN TODAY'S PRIMARY SCHOOLS

Let's talk about that "trainability" and schools. Most people still think of "intelligence" as fixed. Now, I recently read a report on how KIPP schools emphasize the training on some basic skills, such as shared attention, as a needed foundation for good academic performance. So, even if limited in scope, it seems some schools are starting to understand their role in cognitive development. In your experience, are schools fulfilling their roles as "brain gyms", places where young minds get shaped and ready for life?

As a pediatrician working with schools in the Cleveland area since 1985, I have seen all kinds of diseases. For example, I have witnessed the growing incidence of autism spectrum disorders, such as autism and Asperger's. I have also observed how school-work has increasingly become more cognitively demanding, starting with kindergarten.

There is too much pressure on kids as well as their teachers today and a growing number of problems. Yet, I do not see that schools are applying the best knowledge of how minds work. Just as doctors offices are centers of applied medical science, taking the latest advances in medical research and applying them to the medical care of people, schools should be the best place for applied neuroscience, taking the latest advances in cognitive research and applying it to the job of educating minds. Yet, they are not. I can not blame them, given the wide variety of pressures they work under, and the large change in perspective becoming institutes of applied neuroscience would take.

Some readers may be skeptical of the claim that school work is more demanding today than, say, twenty years ago. They may say kids are simply becoming "lazy". What do you say to that?

I have never met a lazy kid. All people want to succeed, in life if not in school. Most children who struggle at school struggle mightily to get adequate grades. It is true that some are more resilient that others. If resilient students fail, they will try ten times harder. The ones that are labeled as "lazy" are typically ashamed of their lack of capacity to deal with demands, and resort to an evasive strategy. They try to avoid the whole situation, to run away.

MEMORY TRAINING IN THE CLASSROOM

You mention a "lack of capacity to deal with demands." Is that gap growing? The equation has two components: capacity and demands. In terms of capacity, the French Education Ministry recently introduced mental arithmetic as part of the curriculum. I remember, as a kid, spending many hours in math class where teachers would require us to perform a progressively complex sequence of mental calculations - which is good training for skills such as working memory. Is memory training coming back into vogue?

Great point. For example, years ago we had to memorize long texts. No matter what the content was, that was a great way to train and build our attention span, working memory, and to devise strategies to learn. Today, there are less opportunities for such memory training in the classroom.

In terms of demands, I can see how complex homework assignments are these days even in third and fourth grades. Kids need to plan and prepare a whole matrix of tasks that require good organizational work to complete. They need to sequence what they do today, tomorrow, and the day after. The major difficulty, for which such young brains may not be fully ready, is to deal with an overwhelming amount of information and demands, and execute.

DEALING WITH ATTENTION DEFICITS IN SCHOOLS

That seems to imply a higher need for good executive functions than years ago. A kid needs to have good working memory to retain, prioritize and sequence much information into actionable plans, and then execute them. From my previous interviews with Dr. Klingberg and Dr. Gibson, we know that a common problem with many kids with diagnosed attention deficits is, indeed, working memory. Can you explain what you see about this in your work with schools?

I am afraid that many schools are too quick to diagnose ADD/ADHD and consider drugs as the only potential intervention. The label itself can be misleading and counterproductive. School psychologists have wonderful expertise in evaluating subject-related problems and describing attention deficit symptoms, but are not trained or asked to complete neuropsychological profiles of a child's cognitive functions.

Up to a point, many kids with attention problems would benefit from educational, not medical, interventions to improve cognitive functions such as working memory. I am seeing it first hand, having used Cogmed Working Memory Training (RoboMemo) with fifteen pre-screened kids. In my practice, eighty percent of students presented a substantive improvement. With fifty percent the results we have seen have been dramatic.

Please give us some examples, so our readers can better understand what working memory is and its role in academic performance and daily life.

Let me give you three vignettes from my clinical experience. All three kids had diagnosed attention deficits and showed clear benefit not only on cognitive functioning but also on AD/HD rating scales.

Patient 1: Eleven year-old boy, very impulsive, even on medication. Did not do homework, constantly forgot chores. After the five week program, he was able to sit down and listen to instructions, engaging in fewer arguments with his parents. He was able to do better mental math for the first time in his life without using his fingers. He found that following school and doing homework was easier and his grades improved dramatically.

Patient 2: Sixteen year-old girl with ADD. She had trouble executing homework, often telling parents she had done it when she really had not. Her parents thought she liked to lie. Yet, when I talked to her, she was clearly more ashamed than dishonest. The working memory training program helped her develop a much improved perception of time. For example, she started to manage her shower time better, being aware of when five minutes had passed-instead of spending thirty minutes in the shower, as before. Her school work improved and her time lying around at home dropped dramatically.

Patient 3: Nineteen year-old boy in college, who often became paralyzed when he was faced with complex challenges. He had a tough time with the cognitive training program, but after a while he started learning new strategies, developing self-confidence, and showing marked improvement. After the program, he could break complex tasks into manageable pieces. His attention deficits appeared to threaten his opportunities in his family business. Since he was unable to keep track of change at the cash register, lines at the business would grow and customers got angry, leaving him out of consideration for key start-up employment in the business. Now he can manage day-to-day challenges such as these, and the door to being part of the family business is open. He can sequence tasks and execute then with a clear plan in mind, without being distracted and losing sight of his plan.

Chapter 4:

Brain Training Software: Profiles, Evaluation Criteria, and our 21 Quick Picks

HIGHLIGHTS

- Different people face different cognitive demands, and have different starting points, so there is no general solution for everyone and everything.
- As in physical fitness, informed consumers and professionals must ask themselves: What are the goals we want to accomplish? What specific cognitive functions are we trying to improve on? In what timeframe? What budget can we spend on this?

The state of the research does not allow for strong "prescriptions" or rankings of products: we want to offer you the best information available today so that you can make better informed decisions on what program, if any, may be worth trying for you, your client, patient or loved-one.

4.1. WHICH EXERCISES ARE MOST RELEVANT?

The first question anyone interested in evaluating products should ask is: Which brain functions do I (or my loved-one or my client) need to train? The answer to this question depends a lot on the situation and goals of the person who will use the training product.

The reasoning is the same as with physical fitness: it is obvious that one need to start training with the goal in mind. Is the goal to train abdominal muscles? Biceps? Cardio capacity? Overall maintenance workout?

If the intended user wants general guidelines to maintain his or her brain health, the overall priorities should be the 4 pillars of brain maintenance: balanced diet, stress management, physical exercise and brain exercise. Novelty, variety and challenge should be incorporated in daily life in a variety of ways.

Age has to be taken in the equation when one wonders what skills need to be trained. As you know the brain changes as we age. Some brain areas, such as the frontal lobes, may need extra workout to increase neuroprotection. The frontal lobes support what scientists call executive functions, which cover abilities such as adapting to new situations and planning. The pathways connecting the frontal lobes to the other brain lobes are very slow to mature and they are typically among the first areas to decline with age. As a consequence, depending on one's age, the training focus may shift from one set of skills to another.

If the intended user is a busy executive, he or she may want to focus on both stress management and train specific brain functions that are part of the skills necessary to accomplish his or her work efficiently. For instance, in the financial domain, Dr. Steenbarger differentiates between short-term and long-term traders. The cognitive abilities needed for both types of traders in order to be successful are different. The goal of short-term traders is to be able to process large amounts of information and quickly see patterns in order to make effective decisions. The underlying cognitive functions are then speed of processing and working memory. In contrast, for long-term traders, analytical skills are the most important.

Useful computer-based brain fitness programs have an initial assessment to determine a current baseline and where it makes most sense to start exercising. From there, the computer constantly checks and updates performance to adjust the level of challenge to ensure that the user is pushed a bit each time.

4.2. SHARPBRAINS' CHECKLIST TO EVALUATE COMPUTER-BASED PROGRAMS

Evaluating the usefulness of computer-based brain fitness programs depends on many factors such as the goals, priorities, starting point, budget, etc of the intended user. There is no general ranking of products that would satisfy everybody. This is why we have developed a Brain Fitness Software Evaluation Checklist. When evaluating a software program we recommend asking the following 10 questions:

1. **Are there scientists, ideally neuropsychologists, and a scientific advisory board behind the program?** Neuropsychologists specialize in measuring and understanding human cognition and brain structure and function.

2. **Are there published, peer-reviewed scientific papers in mainstream scientific and professional journals written by those scientists? How many?** This is important to validate the effectiveness of a particular program.

3. **Does the program tell me what part of my brain or which cognitive skill I am exercising? What are the specific benefits claimed for using this program?** Some programs present the benefits in such an imprecise way that it is impossible to tell if they will have any results or not..."brain exercise" itself is a very vague claim, because activities like gardening or learning a new language provide brain exercise too. You need to see something more specific, like what cognitive or emotional skill that program is aimed at.

4. **Is there an independent assessment to measure my progress?** The question is whether the improvement experienced in the program will transfer into real life. To know if such transfer happened we need assessments that are distinct from the exercises themselves.

5. **Is it a structured program with guidance on how many hours per week and days per week to use it?** Brain exercise is not a

magic pill. You have to do the exercises in order to benefit, so you need clarity on the effort required.

6. **Do the exercises vary and teach me something new?** The only way to exercise important parts of our brain is by tackling novel challenges.

7. **Does the program challenge and motivate me, or does it feel like it would become easy once I learned it?** Good brain exercise requires increasing levels of difficulty and challenge.

8. **Does the program fit my personal goals?** Each individual has different goals/ needs when it comes to brain health. For example, some want to manage anxiety, others to improve short-term memory.

9. **Does the program fit my lifestyle?** Some brain exercise programs have shown good short-term results in research environments but are very intense. Others may be more appropriate for use over time.

10. **Am I ready and willing to do the program, or would it be too stressful?** Excess stress reduces, or may even inhibit, neurogenesis - the creation of new neurons. So, it is important to make sure not to do things that stress us in unhealthy ways.

4.3. MAPPING THE BRAIN TRAINING SOFTWARE LANDSCAPE

There is significant variation around what products are designed to do and around how much evidence there is to back them up. This wide variation is often confusing for customers and even professionals. Out of the hundreds of products out there making brain training claims we include in this guide the ones that have at the very least a well-articulated scientific rationale, a basic level of scientific testing and consumer-usability, and are developed by known organizations which offer professional customer care.

Some companies seem to be betting that the main buying criteria for their products will not be clinical validation, but ease of use and engagement value. Other developers are investing in developing the science that will enable them to make clinical claims, but their products run the risk of being too repetitive and uninspiring for consumer audiences.

The majority of products are sold as software that can be loaded onto a home computer or laptop. Some products can only be used online. There are also devices, such as Nintendo's Brain Age that only work on its DS platform, or Dakim's touch screen computer.

In summary, there are multiple factors to take into consideration when selecting a brain fitness product. These factors range from the level of clinical validation to the user's intended goal.

Each buyer, either consumer or professional, would do well to use the Checklist provided above before purchasing any product. To help you further, we have selected 21 Quick Picks by rating programs against the criteria in the Checklist based on our judgment, the evidence available, and consumer and professional feedback that we have received over the last 2 years.

4.4. TOP 21 QUICK PICKS, BY PURPOSE

The first question to ask as a consumer or professional is, What are my goals or the goal of my client or loved-one? To help you choose products based on your answers to that question we have categorized brain training software based on their purpose: overall brain maintenance, targeted improvement in one specific cognitive domain, and stress management. Note that the products are simply listed by alphabetical order in each table – we have resisted the temptation to rank them because we would be mixing apples with oranges.

Top 8 overall brain maintenance products

The goal of these products is to provide whole brain stimulation. They include a variety of exercises targeting different types of cognitive abilities including memory, attention, language skills, visual skills and reasoning.

They represent an evolution of the classic paper-based options such as crosswords puzzles, word search and Sudoku. They may be more effective than their paper-based cousins for several reasons: (a) they present more novelty, (b) they are more varied, (c) they are usually more challenging and (d) they can be tailored to the user's performance.

Product	Product Type and Target Age	Brain Function	Clinical Validation	Price
Brain Age: Train Your Brain in Minutes a Day and Brain Age 2: More Training in Minutes a Day, by Nintendo	Handheld device (Nintendo DS), all ages	Variety	Very limited	$19.99 for the game, which needs to be played on the Nintendo DS ($129.99).
BrainWare Safari, by Learning Enhancement Corporation	Online, for children	Variety	Low	$349.
FitBrains.com, by Vivity Labs	Online, all ages	Variety	Very limited	All games can be played for free. Paid membership ($9.95/ month, or $79.95/ year) gives access to a variety of community tools.
Happy-neuron.com, by Scientific Brain Training	Online, for adults	Variety	Low	5 free games. Subscription costs $9.95/ month, or $99.95/ year.
Lumosity.com, by Lumos Labs	Online, all ages	Variety	Low	One-week free trial. $9.95/ month, or $79.95/ year afterwards.
MindFit, by CogniFit	Software program, for adults	Variety	Low	$149.
(m)Power, by Dakim	Complete system, including touch-screen computer, for residences	Variety	Low	Around $6-8,000, which includes software, hardware, and services that can be used by up to 12 users in residential settings.

TABLE 6. Products targeting overall brain maintenance.

Top 8 targeted brain workout products

In contrast to whole brain stimulation products, these products focus their efforts on specific cognitive domain such as auditory processing, working memory or visual processing. The goal of all the exercises in each product is to boost performance in the cognitive abilities that are targeted by the product, and closely related ones.

Product Name	Product Type and Target Age	Brain Function	Clinical Validation	Price
Brain Fitness Program Classic, by Posit Science	Software program, for adults	Auditory processing	Medium	$395.
Cogmed JM (children 4-7), RM (ages 7-20) By Cogmed	Software program, for children and adolescents	Working memory	Medium	Around $1,500 which includes the program itself and supervision by a certified clinician.
DriveFit (Golden), by CogniFit	Software program, for older drivers	Assessment and training of variety of driving-related brain functions	Low	$99.
Earobics, by Houghton Mifflin	Software program, for children	Auditory and phonological awareness skills (early literacy skills).	Low-Medium	$59/ user or $299 for a "clinic" version of up to 12 users.
Fast Forword, by Scientific Learning	Family of software-based products, for children	Auditory processing and language-related areas.	Medium	Around $800.
InSight with Cortex, by Posit Science	Software program, for adults	Visual processing	Low-Medium	$395.

IntelliGym, by Applied Cognitive Engineering	Software program, for basketball players	Basketball-specific brain functions (peripheral vision, decision making, situation awareness, attention)	Low	$99 for a personal edition. Several thousand dollars for customized packages for professional teams.
Vision Restoration Therapy, by NovaVision	Software program, for rehabilitation clinics	Vision-related	Medium – High	Several thousand dollars, depending on clinical provider.

TABLE 7. Products focusing on a specific cognitive domain.

Top 5 stress management products

These products are based on biofeedback. As a consequence, they include sensors that measure skin conductivity and/ or heart rate variability, which are associated with physiological stress.

Product name	Product Type and Target Age	Brain Function	Clinical validation	Price
emWave PC Stress Relief, by HeartMath	Software program + biofeedback sensors, all ages	Emotional self-regulation	Low-Medium	$299.
emWave Personal Stress Reliever, by HeartMath	Handheld device, all ages	Emotional self-regulation	Low	$199.

Journey Wild Divine: the Passage, by Wild Divine	Software program + biofeedback sensors, all ages	Emotional self-regulation	Very limited	$159.95.
RESPeRATE, by InterCure Ltd	Medical device, adults	Emotional self-regulation	Medium-High	$299.95.
StressEraser, by Helicor	Handheld device, adults	Emotional self-regulation	Low-Medium	$179.

TABLE 8. Products for stress management.

4.5. PRODUCTS DESCRIPTION AND HIGHLIGHTS

The above Top 21 Quick Picks section categorized products based on their purpose. In the following section we provide more information on each specific product. The categorization by purpose used for the Quick Picks is used again to facilitate your search for specific products.

Overall brain maintenance products

BRAIN AGE

www.brainage.com

The handheld device provides good fun at low cost. It is a worthy product for anyone who is not spending hours in other type of videogames, and for whom the alternative would be doing more crossword puzzles or sudoku.

Nintendo is not conducting any research and does not claim any scientifically proven effects of using the game. Rather, the program announces to users that it was "inspired by" Dr. Kawashima's publications.

BRAINWARE SAFARI

www.brainwareforyou.com

This program is designed to train 41 cognitive skills among kids aged 6-12 in a multimedia gaming format. A small pilot study has shown promising results.

FITBRAINS.COM

www.fitbrains.com

The games were designed with the input from neuropsychologist Dr. Paul Nussbaum. The subscription gives access to tools for continued motivation and engagement, such as competitions, collaborative games, and frequent feedback.

This product may constitute a good alternative to mainstream casual games.

HAPPY-NEURON.COM

www.happy-neuron.com

Scientific Brain Training (SBT)'s scientific advisory board is led by Dr. Bernard Croisile. SBT has agreements with AARP, Prevention.com and others to power their Brain Games section, so you can check them out there for free. In addition to the on-line games, several CD-Rom based games are offered.

This product includes the largest variety of games (35), including 5 ready for the Nintendo Wii.

LUMOSITY.COM

www.lumosity.com

Lumos Labs' scientific advisory board is composed by researchers at top universities.

Their website presents an engaging online experience. It may provide a good value-per-dollar for anyone with high-speed Internet access and a general "mental sharpening" goal.

The only clinical validation consists in a small, unpublished trial that was presented at the Society for Neuroscience Conference in 2006. The company is currently focusing its research on the effect on cognitive rehabilitation following chemotherapy.

MINDFIT

www.e-mindfitness.com

This is the only software with an embedded stand-alone and comprehensive assessment of 14 different cognitive skills, used to tailor the program to the user's needs.

Clinical validation is ongoing: several studies have been conducted but none have been published so far. One study was presented at a 2007 Alzheimer's Conference in Salzburg, Austria.

This product was endorsed by Dr. Susan Greenfield, Director of the Royal Institution in the UK, and is the co-winner of the 2007 American Society on Aging's Business and Aging Award.

(M)POWER

www.dakim.com

Dakim's scientific advisory board is led by Dr. Gary Small.

This product is specially designed for retirement communities and people not familiarized with computers. It includes a touch-screen system and the content is fun.

Targeted brain workout products

BRAIN FITNESS CLASSIC BY POSIT SCIENCE

www.positscience.com/products

This product is best for adults over 60 who feel it takes them longer to follow conversations, especially in noisy environments. It is available both for PC and Mac. It is very demanding.

Posit Science's scientific advisory board is led by Dr. Michael Merzenich. In 2006, Dr. Merzenich and colleagues published a randomized controlled trial using the classic program in the Proceedings of the National Academy of Sciences (PNAS). Further research is under way with the IMPACT study: the initial (yet unpublished) results are promising. Multiple unpublished studies are looking at a variety of applications, from healthy aging to neurological side effects of chemotherapy, Mild Cognitive Impairment, HIV-related, schizophrenia.

The classic Posit Science program is the co-winner of the 2007 American Society on Aging's Business and Aging Award. It is featured on PBS specials on Brain Fitness & Neuroplasticity and in several recent books.

COGMED WORKING MEMORY TRAINING

www.cogmed.com

This product is typically used in clinical settings to help people with attention deficits or individuals undergoing neuropsychological rehabilitation. However, it has not been yet cleared by FDA for any therapeutic application.

Cogmed was founded by Dr. Torkel Klingberg. There are several clinical trials under way by independent researchers. Dr. Klingberg published a randomized controlled trial with children with attention deficits in the Journal of the American Academy of Child and Adolescent Psychiatry (2005), and several related studies in a variety of respected journals.

DRIVEFIT (GOLDEN DRIVEFIT)

www.e-mindfitness.com

This product is best for older adults who want to improve driving-related cognitive skills, Clinical validation is low. Nonetheless, with the British School of Motoring, DriveFit won the prestigious Prince Michael Road Safety Award for a similar product focused on teenagers.

EAROBICS

www.earobics.com

This product is best to help students in pre-K through third grade develop early literacy skills.

The What Works Clearinghouse, maintained by the US Department of Education, considers the extent of evidence for Earobics to be small for both alphabetics and fluency.

FASTFORWORD

www.scilearn.com

Fast Forword has been shown to be an effective intervention for dyslexic students who struggle with the specific cognitive skills that the program trains (auditory and phonological skills). According to the What Works Clearinghouse database, maintained by the Department of Education, the fit may be less clear for students who are not dyslexic.

The software is very demanding and usually requires parents' or school supervision for compliance.

INSIGHT

www.positscience.com/products

This product is best for adults over 50 who notice loss of concentration and attention abilities while doing complex tasks, such as driving.

One of the five exercises included in the program, the UFOV (Useful Field of View) exercise, is based on many previous scientific studies (See interview with Dr. Elizabeth Zelinski in Chapter 2). The other four exercises have not been tested before.

INTELLIGYM

www.intelligym.com

This product is best for committed players and teams. It should be considered as a serious workout, not a game.

Dr. Daniel Gopher acts as an advisor to Applied Cognitive Engineering. IntelliGym is used by prestigious NCAA basketball teams, such as Kentucky, Memphis, Florida, Kansas.

VISION RESTORATION THERAPY

www.novavision.com

This product obtained 510(k) clearance FDA clearance in April 2003 for patients recovering from stroke or traumatic brain injury. It constitutes a very expensive intervention. Clinical validation is based on two published controlled trials.

Stress management products

EMWAVE

The PC Stress Relief (software program and biofeedback sensors, www.emwavepc.com) can be used both by individuals and by professionals (like psychologists or educators) who can use the program with multiple users. The product has a New Age feel that can sometimes gets in the way.

The Personal Stress Reliever (handheld device, www.emwave.com) is easy-to-use on the go. It is currently popular with nurses and golf players.

JOURNEY WILD DIVINE

www.wilddivine.com

This product is best for people looking to learn and explore in a gaming environment. It combines fun with benefits and presents a New Age look-and-feel. It can be considered more as a game than a training product.

RESPERATE

www.resperate.com

This product is a portable medical device that has been shown to help lower blood pressure. Recommended use is 15 minutes a day, several times a week.

STRESSERASER

www.stresseraser.com

This product is a no-frills biofeedback device, popular with busy professionals and executives. It has limited published clinical evidence, but a high-quality Scientific Advisory Board.

Chapter 5.
A Growing Range of Applications

Brain training has more current and future applications than meet the eye. The same way there are many reasons to exercise our bodies (run in a marathon, stay in shape, lose weight, become an Olympian, have strong abdominal muscles, etc.), there are many reasons to exercise our brains. In this chapter, we review a few current and future applications of brain training, such as the use of brain training in retirement communities, at school or in the clinical world.

5.1. HEALTHY AGING

If you were born between 1946 and 1964 you are probably going to work and live longer than any previous generation. It is also very likely that you have had some experience with Alzheimer's disease or other types of dementia either through a loved one, a client or a patient.

This is why more and more adults are currently eager to try new approaches to reduce the rate and impact of cognitive decline. They want to "train their brains" using high tech games that go beyond the traditional crossword puzzles.

5.2. BRAIN FITNESS CENTERS IN RESIDENTIAL FACILITIES

In-house "brain fitness centers" are becoming more common in retirement communities, nursing homes, and continuing care retirement communities

(CCRCs) around the country. These centers are usually composed of several computers and a trained facilitator and they complement existing wellness, social and enrichment activities.

Based on multiple interviews with industry experts and program manufacturers, we estimate that over 600 communities in the US, mostly independent living and CCRCs, already offer computerized brain fitness programs to their residents. Not a week goes by without at least one such community issuing a press release announcing the use of these programs.

However there are equal amounts of interest and confusion among executives and professionals thinking about adding computer-based cognitive exercise products to their mix of health and wellness activities. This is why we developed the Evaluation Checklist that follows, to help seniors housing environments select programs.

SHARPBRAINS CHECKLIST FOR BRAIN FITNESS CENTERS IN SENIORS HOUSING

1. **Early users:** Who among our residents is ready and willing to do the program? How are they reacting to the pilot testing of the program?
2. **Cognitive benefits:** What are the specific benefits claimed for using this program? Under what scenario of use (how many hours/week, how many weeks)? What specific cognitive skill(s) does the program train? How will we measure progress?
3. **Return on investment:** What are our key objectives, and how will we independently measure the progress due to this program so we can evaluate the business case to expand, maintain, or change course?
4. **Appropriate challenge**: Do the exercises adjust to the individual and continually vary and challenge residents at an appropriate pace?
5. **Scientific credentials**: Are there scientists, ideally neuropsychologists, behind the program? Is there a clearly defined and credible scientific advisory board? Are there any published, peer-reviewed scientific papers?
6. **Product roadmap**: What is the product roadmap for this company? What is the company developing and planning to offer next year, and in 2–3 years?

7. **Technical requirements**: What are the technical requirements needed to successfully deploy and maintain the program? Does it require an Internet connection? Who will help solve potential glitches?

8. **Staff training**: What type of training will my staff need, and who will provide it?

9. **Total cost of ownership**: What may be the total cost of ownership over the next 3–5 years if we go with this vendor: upfront fees, ongoing fees, hardware, software, training and support fees, cost of additional modules and staff time? How many residents will likely end up using the system, and therefore what is the Cost of Ownership per User?

10. **References**: What similar communities have used this specific program? What proportion of their residents uses it regularly? What benefits have they measured and observed in their residents, and as a community? Is the use of the program growing, or is it flat or declining?

5.3. COGNITIVE ASSESSMENTS

Many studies have shown that when the right group of people uses the right tool, significant benefits can occur. The question then becomes, "What assessments may help pinpoint who may benefit from what type of training, and set up objective, independent baselines for cognitive performance over time?"

Users of brain fitness products will need assessments to identify cognitive bottlenecks, that is, the cognitive skills that constrain the others and that, if improved, can have a positive impact on other functions. The development of inexpensive and widely available, yet valid and reliable, cognitive assessments will then be critical to the mainstream growth of the brain fitness field.

Most assessments today that require the participation of trained professionals are expensive and present limited scalability. A major issue in the use and refinement of cognitive training tools for the appropriate groups today and in the future is the time and economic investment involved in mostly face-to-face neuropsychological assessments.

To address this issue, a number of fully-automated computer-based cognitive assessments are being used more frequently in large-scale clinical trials, helping pharmaceutical companies identify and evaluate potential cognitive effects of drugs. The primary goal behind the design of these neurocognitive batteries is not to diagnose individual patients, but to measure cognition with enough reliability and validity to show objective baselines and any changes relative to this baseline in large subject samples.

This may well open the way for such assessments to be made available for a wider array of consumer uses. Potentially, these assessments could be repurposed to help establish a cognitive baseline, assess mental functioning before and after clinical conditions, track the consequences of aging, identify priorities for cognitive training, and measure progress independent from the training itself in individual patients and healthy individuals.

5.4. PROGRAMS TO IMPROVE DRIVING SKILLS

As drivers get older a number of cognitive problems can get in the way of safe driving.

The insurance company Allstate recently started a research study to evaluate innovative ways to alleviate this problem. Allstate is now offering for free the InSight program (a Posit Science program) to several thousand 50-75 year-old, auto policy-holders in Pennsylvania, as well as to some potential clients. They recommend participants to devote at least 10 hours to the training exercises. They expect the software exercises to reduce risky driving maneuvers and improve stopping distance. The goal is to see whether computerized brain training can help reduce the number of accidents in the group participating in the exercises compared to the group of policy-holders who are not. InSight focuses mostly on visual processing but prior studies, conducted by Dr. Jerri Edwards (whose interview you can find at the end of this chapter) have shown that computerized program focusing on visual awareness can indeed improve driving skills.

An increasing number of traffic schools in Europe and Canada, as well as US companies that employ large numbers of drivers, are adding a new tool to their assessment and training toolkit: the DriveFit technology, developed by CogniFit. This program was awarded the prestigious Prince Michael International Award for Road Safety for its 'outstanding contribution to road safety' in the UK. DriveFit is a suite of programs aimed at helping to assess and build the cognitive, psychomotor and personality skills needed by novice, senior and fleet drivers. The product is distributed by country-specific agreements with chains of traffic schools, such as Young Drivers of Canada (over 100 centers) and the British School of Motoring (BSM) in the UK (with 107 centers).

According to non-published research from driving training experts at the British School of Motoring, learners who trained with MAP (Mental Alertness Programme, developed by CogniFit for BSM, building on DriveFit) recorded a 16 percent higher pass rate (of the exam required to obtain a driving license) than ones who did not use the program.

5.5. BRAIN DISORDERS

Increasingly, there are a variety of clinical conditions for which non-invasive, computerized cognitive training programs can play a role both as first line interventions and post diagnosis to complement existing treatments. In conditions such as stroke, traumatic brain injury, and attention deficits disorders some programs are getting traction and building practitioner networks.

Stroke / Traumatic Brain Injury

For many years, neuropsychologists have used cognitive rehabilitation to help patients suffering from strokes (cerebrovascular accident or CVA) and traumatic brain injury (TBI). Cognitive rehabilitation aims at establishing brain functional changes by (a) restructuring previously learned behaviors, and (b) establishing new cognitive patterns thanks to compensatory mechanisms. It offers retraining in the ability to think, use judgment, make decisions, as well as to rehabilitate verbal and visuo-spatial skills, memory, attention, and other functions which may suffer following CVA or TBI. Along with other tools, cognitive exercises, including computer-assisted strategies are used during the training. The development and validation of new brain training software is thus important in this area.

Two recent, comprehensive literature reviews by Cicerone (2000, 2005) on evidence based cognitive rehabilitation found out that cognitive rehabilitation provides significant benefit when compared with alternative treatments. The analysis covered 47 treatment comparisons representing 1801 patients.

NovaVision is an example of a computerized program used in the clinical field. NovaVision obtained 510(k) clearance by the FDA in April 2003 for its "Vision Restoration Therapy." The intended use of this program is the "diagnosis and improvement of visual functions in patients with impaired vision that may have resulted from stroke, trauma, inflammation, surgical removal of brain tumors or brain surgery." Note that NovaVision's product had received prior clinical validation. In 1998, in *Nature Medicine*, Kasten and colleagues showed that vision can be improved in patients with visual-field defects thanks to the repetitive computerized stimulation of the visual field provided by NovaVision's product.

Recent world events will soon shape the advances made in this area. Indeed, in 2007, given the high rates of Iraq War veterans with TBI (estimated at above 10 percent), Congress authorized an appropriation of close to $20m to conduct research and develop applications to diagnose and treat soldiers with TBI.

Attention deficit disorders

A Center for Disease Control report (2007) estimated that, in 2003, 4.4 million youth between four and seventeen years old lived with diagnosed Attention Deficit Hyperactivity Disorder (ADHD), and 2.5 million of them were being treated for this condition with drugs.

The view of a respected researcher in the field, Dr. Russell Barkley, is gaining ground. Dr. Barkley argues that the main deficit associated with ADHD is the failure to develop the capacity for self-regulation or self control. As a result, specific and important brain processes and functions fail to develop in an optimal way. Dr. Barkley highlights the following four problem areas: working memory, internalization of speech, sense of time, and goal directed behavior.

Following the publication in the *Journal of the American Academy of Child and Adolescent Psychiatry* of a double-blind controlled clinical trial that showed how working memory training improved a number of non-trained cognitive skills and alleviated behavioral symptoms in children with ADD/ADHD (Klingberg et al, 2005), a network of US clinicians are offering Cogmed's working memory training.

According to Dr. Arthur Lavin, many school psychologists may be too quick to diagnose ADD/ADHD. This can be misleading and even counterproductive for some children. In addition, it is often the case that drugs are considered as the only potential intervention. Dr Lavin believes that "Up to a point, many kids with attention problems would benefit from educational, not medical, interventions to improve cognitive functions such as working memory." (see Dr. Lavin's interview at the end of Chapter 3)

5.6. SCHOOLS

One of the first computer-based cognitive training programs ever commercialized was created for the K12 education segment. The product, called Fast Forword, was launched by Scientific Learning Corporation (SCIL) in 1997. It focused on helping students with dyslexia and was distributed through clinical channels.

Given the pressures on academic results intensified by the Bush administration's No Child Left Behind (NCLB) Act of 2001, school districts have invested heavily in programs that directly address academic disciplines such as math and reading. Cognitive training, in comparison, suffers given its "indirect" relationship to those academic disciplines. Although it may be logical to assume that if a program helps a child improve underlying reading-related cognitive abilities that the program will ultimately help the child be a better reader, clinical research has not yet been conducted to solidify this critical link beyond the small percentage of kids with severe dyslexia problems.

In 2002, the U.S. Department of Education's Institute of Education Sciences established the What Works Clearinghouse (WWC) to provide the education community and the public with a centralized and trusted source of scientific evidence of what works in education. So far, two computerized cognitive training programs have merited inclusion in the What Works Clearinghouse: Scientific Learning's Fast Forword and Houghton Mifflin's Earobics.

In order to include a program in the Clearinghouse, review teams comb through the scientific literature and analyze the appropriate research evidence supporting specific educational interventions. The primary goal is to clarify the evidence of causal validity in existing studies, categorizing them in one of three ways:

- "Meets Evidence Standards" for randomized controlled trials and regression discontinuity studies that provide the strongest evidence of causal validity,
- "Meets Evidence Standards with Reservations" for quasi-experimental studies; randomized controlled trials that have problems with randomization, attrition, or disruption; and regression discontinuity designs that have problems with attrition or disruption, or
- "Does Not Meet Evidence Screens" for studies that do not provide strong evidence of causal validity.

Based on the studies that pass this screening and are categorized as either "meets evidence standards" or "meets evidence standards with reservations," the What Works Clearinghouse issues a report that summarizes the intervention and its evidence-based results. This report can be found on the What Works Clearinghouse website (http://ies.ed.gov/ncee/wwc/).

5.7. INSURANCE COMPANIES

Given the expected growth of Alzheimer's disease across the aging US population and the cost of patient care, insurance companies have a strong interest in reducing the rate of cognitive decline, delaying the onset of Mild Cognitive Decline and Alzheimer's symptoms and slowing the progression of the disease once it appears.

Some insurance pioneers such as Humana and MetLife are experimenting with offering brain fitness programs and providing incentives to their members to live healthier lifestyles. In 2006 and 2007, Humana rolled out a multi-million dollar agreement with Posit Science to offer Posit's program for free or at reduced rates to its Medicare members.

Insurance companies are among the leaders in disseminating information about the benefits of healthy brain habits. In 2005, MetLife produced and distributed a brochure on Ten Tips for Maintaining a Healthy Brain.

Despite the lack of product-specific long-term efficacy results, insurers see the value of adding a brain component to wellness and prevention initiatives from a member recruitment and loyalty point of view.

5.8. INTERVIEWS:

- Dr. Daniel Gopher: Applications for computer-based cognitive simulations.
- Dr. David Rabiner: Brain exercise implications for children with ADD/ADHD.
- Dr. Torkel Klingberg: Expanding working memory for children with ADD/ADHD.
- Dr. Jerri Edwards: Improving driving skills.

Interview with Dr. Daniel Gopher – Applications of computer-based cognitive simulations.

BACKGROUND:

Dr. Daniel Gopher is one of the world's leading figures in the field of cognitive training. He is a fellow of the U.S. Human Factors and Ergonomics Society and the International Ergonomics Association. He is a Professor of Cognitive Psychology and Human Factors Engineering and Director of the Research Center for Work Safety at Israel's Technion Institute of Science.

During his forty year career, he has held a variety of scientific and academic positions, such as acting Head of the Research Unit of the Military Personnel Division in Israel, Associate Editor of the *European Journal of Cognitive Psychology*, member of the Editorial Boards of *Acta Psychologica*, the *International Journal of Human-Computer Interaction*, and *Psychology*. He published an award-winning article on how flight skills transferred from computer games to real life.

Dr. Gopher has developed innovative medical systems that assess the nature and causes of human error in medical work and redesign medical work environments to improve safety and efficiency. He has also developed work safety systems including methods and models for the analysis of human factors, ergonomics, safety and health problems at the individual, team and plant level.

HIGHLIGHTS:

- Cognitive performance can be substantially improved with proper training. It is not rigidly constrained by innate, fixed abilities.
- To effectively transfer skills from training to reality, a training program needs to ensure cognitive fidelity, rather than physical fidelity which is more common.

CURRENT RESEARCH

What are you currently working on?

Since 1980, I have been the Director of the Research Center for Work Safety and Human Engineering, an interdisciplinary research center which involves thirty researchers from five Technion faculties and eighty graduate students, who work in seven laboratories. I also act as Scientific Advisor for ACE's *Intelligym* and am involved in a new integrative research project labeled "Skills-Multimodal Interfaces for the Capturing and Transfer of Skills," directed to facilitate and improve the acquisition and transfer of skills through the development of innovative virtual-reality multimodal interfaces. This is an initiative supported by the European Commission with fifteen industry and university research partners, from nine countries.

What are your current research interests?

My main interest has been how to expand the limits of human attention, information processing and response capabilities which are critical in complex, real time decision making, high demand tasks such as flying a military jet or playing professional basketball. Using a tennis analogy, my goal has been, and is, how to help develop many Wimbledon-like champions each with his/her own style, but performing at maximum capacity to succeed in various environments.

EFFECTIVE SKILLS TRANSFER: FROM PROGRAMS TO DAILY LIFE

What does your research tell us about what makes a skills training program most effective?

What research over the last fifteen to twenty years has shown is that cognition, or what we call thinking and performance, is really a set of skills that we can train systematically. And that computer-based cognitive trainers or "cognitive simulations" are the most effective and efficient way to do so.

This is an important point, so let me emphasize it. What we have discovered is that a key factor for an effective transfer from training environment to reality is that the training program ensures cognitive fidelity, that is, it should faithfully represent the mental demands that happen in the real world. Traditional approaches tend to focus instead on physical fidelity, which may seem more intuitive, but is less effective and harder to achieve. They are also less efficient, given costs involved in creating expensive physical simulators that faithfully replicate, let's say, a whole military helicopter or just a significant part of it.

In the 2007 Serious Games Summit, we saw a number of simulations for military training that try to be as realistic as possible. Are you saying that they may not be the best approach for training?

The need for physical fidelity is not based on research, at least for the type of high performance training we are talking about. In fact, a simple environment may be better in that it does not create the illusion of reality.

Simulations can be very expensive and complex, sometimes even costing as much as the real thing, which limits the access to training. Not only that, but the whole effort may be futile, given that some important features can not be replicated (such as gravitation free tilted or inverted flight), and even result in negative transfer, because learners pick up on specific training features or sensations that do not exist in the real situation.

What are the main studies you have conducted on skills transfer from computer programs?

In this field of work, I would mention two. In one, which constituted the basis for the 1994 paper, we showed that ten hours of training for flight cadets in an attention trainer instantiated as a computer game – *Space Fortress* – resulted in thirty percent improvement in flight performance. The results led the trainer to be integrated into the regular training program of the flight school. It was used in the training of hundreds of flight cadets for several years.

In the other study, sponsored by NASA, we compared the results of the cognitive trainer versus a sophisticated, pictorial and high level graphic and physical fidelity-based computer simulation of a Blackhawk helicopter. The result: the *Space Fortress* cognitive trainer was very successful in improving performance, while the alternative was not.

APPLYING COMPUTER-BASED COGNITIVE SIMULATIONS TO REAL LIFE

What have been to date the main applications of your computer-based cognitive simulations?

In summary, I would say:

- Flying high-performance airplanes – in ten hours, we showed an increase in thirty percent flight performance
- Flying with HMD (helmet mounted displays)
- Touch-typing skills
- Teaching old adults to cope with high workload attention demands
- Developing Basketball "game intelligence" for professional players, to improve the performance of individuals and teams

Talk to us about the basketball example. I am sure many readers will find that fascinating.

I served as a scientific advisor to ACE, which developed the program called *Intelligym*. Although the context is different, the approach and basic principles are the same as those of developing a trainer for the task of flying a high performance jet airplane.

First, one needs to analyze what cognitive skills are involved in playing at top level, and then develop a computer-based cognitive simulation that trains those skills. What most people do not realize is that top players are not born top players. We are not just talking about instincts. We are talking about skills that can be trained.

What have the results of the ACE Intelligym been for basketball players so far?

First, let me say that the company has had to overcome huge cultural barriers to get adoption by a good number of university teams and some NBA players. Coaches see the value of this tool very quickly, but administrators are harder to convince in the beginning.

We have seen that the basketball teams and individuals using *Intelligym* have improved their performance significantly. From the cognitive training, or skill development point of view, we have seen that players improve their positional awareness – of themselves, their team mates and opponents – and their ability to predict what is going on in the game. Players are also able to make fast and good decisions. Players quickly develop attention allocation strategies that enable them to better participate in the game, and also improve their spatial orientation.

LESSONS LEARNED

Please summarize your research findings across all these examples and fields, and how you see the field evolving.

In short, I'd summarize by saying that cognitive performance can be substantially improved with proper training. It is not rigidly constrained by innate, fixed abilities. Cognitive task analysis enables us to extract major cognitive skills involved in any task. Attention control and attention allocation strategies are critical determinants in performing at top level in complex, real time decision making environments. Those skills, and other associated ones, can be improved through training. Research shows that stand alone, inexpensive, PC-based training is effective to transfer and generalize performance. The key to success is to ensure cognitive fidelity, this is, that the cognitive demands in training resemble those of the real life task.

I can think of many other applications. Probably currency and options traders would benefit from a system like this. Now, we will need to increase awareness, and will need to find champions willing to take risks. The cognitive simulation approach is less intuitive than traditional ones.

Professor Wayne Shebilske, at Wright State University Psychology department, is conducting additional research.

For readers who may be interested in more specific details about your specific approach to cognitive training, could you give us some of your personal lessons learned?

There are different types of cognitive training. The one we have specialized in focuses on the development of attention control and attention allocation strategies, which are bottlenecks in some high performing, high mental workload environments. Our approach is called Emphasis Change Protocol and is based on the introduction of systematic variability in training, while maintaining the overall task intact. We just change the emphasis on sub-components of a complex task during performance. In our research, this has proven to be the most effective way to train attention management skills, task switching and control processes, such as the ability to initiate, coordinate, synchronize and regulate goal-directed behavior.

This "whole task" approach increases transfer and adaptation capabilities versus traditional part task training, which decomposes the complex task and trains elements in isolation. However, whole task training is harder at the beginning. There is slower progress at early stages of training.

Other principles we use, based on our and others' literature, is the need for intermittent schedules of feedback. This has been shown to help with retention and transfer (at the cost of making learning slower).

Another principle we use is encouragement to explore alternatives to reach a general optimum. This exploration is important: we want to help the user find a flexible, and personal, best match between his/her abilities and the task demands. Coming back to the tennis example, we know that McEnroe and Boris Becker have different styles; but both are Wimbledon winners. We want to make sure the user increases sensitivity to real time changes in the environment and expands his or her ability to cope with them.

Interview with Dr. David Rabiner – Brain exercise implications for children with ADD/ADHD.

BACKGROUND:

Dr. David Rabiner is a Senior Research Scientist and the Director of Psychology and Neuroscience Undergraduate Studies at Duke University. He is an advocate for children and adults with ADD/ADHD.

HIGHLIGHTS:

- Attention and working memory can be developed and improved with practice.
- Parents of children with ADHD should make informed decisions by researching the available evidence backing-up or not the interventions.

CURRENT RESEARCH

What are your main research interests?

In summary, I will say that my long standing interests have been how to improve the quality of care received by children with ADD/ADHD and how to ensure a positive relationship between children's social experience and their social cognitive functioning. One of my first ADD/ADHD-related projects was a National Institute of Mental Health-funded grant to assist primary care pediatricians in providing more evidence-based methods for evaluating and treating children with ADHD.

Right now I am an investigator on two research studies. In one, funded by the National Institute of Mental Health, we are conducting a longitudinal study of a large, community-based sample of youth with ADD/ADHD, and tracking their academic, clinical and behavioral performance over six to seven years.

The other one is a three years grant by the Department of Education to evaluate how computer-based programs can help kids with ADD/ADHD. We are analyzing the impact of two types of programs: a) Captain's Log, which is a cognitive training program, and b) curriculum-based programs such as Riverdeep's Destination Reading and Math.

When will we start to see results from those studies?

For the Mental Health longitudinal one, you may have to wait four to five years to see the first papers. For the Department of Education one, some preliminary results will be published in 2008.

COGNITIVE TRAINING APPLICATIONS FOR ADD/ADHD

What are the cognitive training applications that can help people with ADD/ADHD?

Cognitive training rests on solid premises, and some programs already have very promising research results. Cognitive areas, such as attention, or working memory, can be conceptualized as skills. There is growing evidence that like other kinds of skills, they can be developed and improved with concerted practice.

Two of the most promising areas are neurofeedback, which is starting to present good research results, and working memory training, with research led by Dr. Torkel Klingberg.

When Dr. Mark Katz and I met with some school superintendents, he stressed that "attention deficit" is being reframed by the research community as "executive function deficit". The bottleneck or problem is not attention itself, but reliable and self-directed capacity to execute. Can you please elaborate?

Dr. Russell Barkley, Research Professor of Psychiatry at SUNY Medical University and Clinical Professor of Psychiatry at the Medical University of South Carolina, has been a key advocate for this view. Several years ago he published a comprehensive theory of ADHD in which he argues that the core problem is a deficit in "behavior inhibition", and that this deficit interferes with the normal development of important executive functions.

In this theory, the behavioral symptoms that are currently used to diagnose ADHD – including inattention – reflect these underlying executive functioning deficits. There certainly is substantial evidence that individuals with ADHD perform more poorly than others – as a group – on a number of executive functioning tasks that require planning, organizational skills, inhibiting responses (as assessed through tasks such as the Stroop test), decision making, working memory and other frontal lobe executive functions. His theory is generating a significant amount of research and it is likely that our conceptualization of ADHD will continue to evolve in response to new findings.

I understand that Dr. Barbara Ingersoll and you co-led a panel at the 2006 Children and Adults with Attention-Deficit/Hyperactivity Disorder (CHADD) Conference, what was the topic?

The title was "New and Complementary Approaches to the Assessment and Treatment of AD/HD." We provided an overview and update of research on complementary approaches to the evaluation and treatment of AD/HD, including the use of Quantitative EEG (QEEG) as part of a comprehensive evaluation for AD/HD, current research pertaining to neurofeedback, and computerized training of working memory as treatments for AD/HD. We also highlighted the rationale and need for new evidence-based approaches to evaluation and treatment.

ADVICE FOR PARENTS OF KIDS WITH ADD/ADHD

Cogmed's Dr. Torkel Klingberg also presented at the 2006 CHADD conference his research on working memory training results in a panel called "Computerized Training of Working Memory in Children with ADHD." What do you recommend that parents do when they are looking for new interventions for their children with ADD/ADHD? How can they navigate through the multiple companies, centers and programs making a variety of claims?

This is a very relevant question. Parents are always looking for ways to help their children. Not only that. Adults with ADD/ADHD are also a very self-motivated group. However, there have been a number of disappointments. I would recommend that parents discuss new interventions with their pediatricians, and also make informed decisions that include reading peer-reviewed publications, or at the very least make themselves aware of what specific interventions have published results in respectable journals.

How can parents, and anyone who is not a scientist, access those publications you mention?

There are different ways. One, they can search for papers in PubMed. Sometimes the papers themselves are not available in PubMed, but the summaries, abstracts, are. If they want to read the whole article, they can go to any university libraries with free access to Medline.

For people who may not want to read the research papers, but be informed of the highlights of new research developments, I launched Attention Research Update, a free monthly newsletter that helps parents, professionals, and educators stay informed about important new research on ADD/ADHD.

Interview with Dr. Torkel Klingberg – Expanding working memory for children with ADD/ADHD.

BACKGROUND:

Dr. Torkel Klingberg is the Director of the Developmental Cognitive Neuroscience Lab at Karolinska Institute which is part of the Stockholm Brain Institute. Dr. Klingberg has published numerous papers in peer-reviewed publications such as the Journal of the American Academy of Child & Adolescent Psychiatry, Journal of Cognitive Neuroscience, and Nature Neuroscience on topics including the effect of working memory training itself and in combination with medication on school performance.

HIGHLIGHTS:

- Working memory training can help children with attention deficits.
- We may be at the beginning of a new era of computerized training with a wide range of applications.

RESEARCH ON WORKING MEMORY TRAINING

What type of research does your Developmental Cognitive Neuroscience Lab at the Karolinska Institute focus on?

The lab is addressing the questions of development and plasticity of working memory. We do that through several techniques, such as fMRI, diffusion tensor imaging to look at myelination of white matter in the brain, neural network models of working memory, and behavioral studies. In addition, I am a scientific advisor for Cogmed, the company that developed and commercializes RoboMemo.

What are the highlights of your research on the effect of working memory?

Our paper from 2004 in *Nature Neuroscience*, on the effect of working memory training on brain activity, and the 2005 randomized, controlled clinical trial on the impact of working memory training specifically in kids with ADD/ADHD, have caught the most public attention.

My other research concerns the neural basis for development and plasticity of cognitive functions during childhood, in particular the development of attention and working memory.

In short, I would say that we have shown that working memory can be improved by training and that such training helps people with attention deficits and it also improves reasoning ability overall.

What are the everyday life effects of working memory training for a child with attention deficits?

When looking at the 1,200 children who have trained in Cogmed's Stockholm Clinic, the most common effects are sustained attention, better impulse control, and improved learning ability. Parents often report that their children perform better in school and are able to keep up a coherent conversation more easily after training. Being able to hold back impulses, such as anger outbursts, and keeping better track of one's things are other everyday life benefits.

How are you making the program available?

All rights are with Cogmed, which is making this available in Sweden and started to offer this to selected clinics in the US in 2006.

FUTURE OF BRAIN FITNESS PROGRAMS AND COGNITIVE TRAINING

What do you expect that we will learn over the next five years or so in the field of brain fitness programs and cognitive training?

I think that we are seeing the beginning of a new era of computerized training for a wide range of applications.

Our studies have mostly been aimed at individuals with visible problems of inattention; but, there is a wider zone concerning what you define as attention problems. We will see how Cogmed can help a larger part of the population in improving cognitive function.

Interview with Dr. Jerri Edwards – Improving driving skills.

BACKGROUND:

Dr. Jerri Edwards is an Associate Professor at University of South Florida's School of Aging Studies and Co-Investigator of the influential ACTIVE study. Dr. Edwards was trained by Dr. Karlene K. Ball, and her research is aimed at discovering how cognitive abilities can be maintained and even enhanced with advancing age.

HIGHLIGHTS:

- Speed of processing can be improved and a significant portion of that improvement stays even after five years.
- Faster speed-of-processing seem to enable adults to react better to unexpected events that require a fast response and to reduce by 40 percent the number of dangerous maneuvers on real roads.

RESEARCH INTERESTS

Please explain to our readers your main research areas.

I am particularly interested in how cognitive interventions may help older adults to avoid or at least delay functional difficulties and thereby maintain their independence longer. Much of my work has focused on the functional ability of driving including assessing driving fitness among older adults and remediation of cognitive decline that results in driving difficulties.

Some research questions that interest me include, how can we maintain healthier lives longer? How can training improve cognitive abilities, both to improve those abilities and also to slow-down, or delay, cognitive decline? The specific cognitive ability that I have studied the most is processing speed, which is one of the cognitive skills that decline early on as we age.

RESULTS OF ACTIVE STUDY

Can you explain what cognitive processing speed is and why it is relevant to our daily lives?

Processing speed is mental quickness. Just like a computer with a 486 processor can do a lot of the same things as a computer with a Pentium 4 processor; but it takes much longer. Our minds tend to slow down with age as compared to when we were younger. We can do the same tasks; but it takes more time. Quick speed of processing is important for quick decision making in our daily lives. When you are driving, if something unexpected happens, how quickly can you notice the situation and decide how to react?

Please describe how the ACTIVE trial used the cognitive training program and what the results were found to be when they were published in the Journal of the American Medical Association in December 2006?

I was a co-investigator of the ACTIVE study, a multi-site, controlled study, with thousands of adults over sixty-five, to evaluate the effectiveness of three different cognitive training methods with three different groups:

- The first group used a memory training program including a variety of traditional memory techniques such as mnemonics and the method of loci.
- The second group was trained to learn inductive reasoning skills.
- The third group was exposed to computer-based programs to train processing speed.

All three groups spent the same amount of time in their respective training programs, around two hours a week for five weeks, going through exercises of increasing difficulty. The ACTIVE study was designed to track participants' performance over a number of years. So, after this initial five week intervention, some groups received training booster sessions after one year and again after three years.

Willis and colleagues published the very positive five year results of the ACTIVE study in JAMA at the end of 2006. The most impressive result was that, when tested five years later, the participants in all three types of training had retained a significant percentage of the improvement compared to the control group. But, the results of the group that used a computer-based program to train processing speed showed more pronounced short-term and long-term improvements. Individuals who experienced improved speed of processing also showed better performance on common tasks instrumental in daily life such as quickly finding an item on a crowded pantry shelf and reading medication bottles. They also reacted to road signs more quickly. We found this transfer of training in our prior studies using the training protocol as well.

In short, significant percentages of the participants improved their memory, reasoning and information processing speed across all three methods. The most impressive result was that, when tested five years later, the participants in the computer-based program had less of a decline in the skill they were trained in than did a control group that received no cognitive training.

CLARIFYING THE CONFUSION ABOUT THE VALUE OF BRAIN FITNESS

The results of the ACTIVE study were quite impressive and contributed in large part to the amount of media coverage about brain fitness last year. However, as you have probably seen, there is a good deal of confusion about brain fitness among the media and the public at large. Can you help our readers understand two common questions: 1) Why are new programs better than, say, doing crosswords puzzles?, and 2) Can one really say that these programs can reverse age-related decline?

To answer the first question, I would say that a crossword puzzle is not a form of cognitive training. It can be stimulating, but it is not a form of structured mental exercise that has been shown to improve specific cognitive skills - other than the skill of doing crossword puzzles, of course.

In terms of the second question, it is too early to say whether we can really reverse decline in a permanent way. There are many skills involved and the studies are not long enough to really compare different trajectories. What we can say is that by doing some exercises, one can improve cognitive speed of processing by 146-250 percent, and that a significant portion of that improvement stays even after five years. We cannot say more definitively.

But, I think it is noteworthy to be able to say that in all of the programs tested, the payoff from cognitive training, or what we can call "mental exercise," seemed far greater than we are accustomed to getting from physical exercise. Just imagine if you could say that ten hours of workouts at the gym every day this month was enough to help keep you fit five years from now.

IMPACT OF COGNITIVE TRAINING ON DRIVING A CAR

Another fascinating study that you published as a co-author in Human Factors (2003), applied a computer-based program to improving the driving-related mental skills of older adults. Can you explain that study?

Sure. Our goal was to train what is called the "useful field of view." The useful field of view is a measure of processing speed and visual attention that is critical for driving performance, and one of the areas that declines with age. It has previously been shown that this skill can be improved with training, so we wanted to see what effect it would have on the driving performance of older adults, and whether the training would be more or less effective than a traditional driving simulation course.

For the study, we divided forty-eight adults over fifty-five years old into two intervention groups of twenty-four people each. Each group received twenty hours of training. One group was exposed to a traditional driving simulator, where they learned specific driving behaviors. The other one went through the cognitive training program.

Both groups' driving performance improved right after their respective programs, but most benefits of the driving simulator disappeared by month eighteen. The speed-of-processing intervention helped participants not only improve "useful field of view," the skill that was directly trained, but it also transferred into real-life driving, and the results were sustained after eighteen months. And, by the way, the evaluation was as real as one can imagine: a fourteen mile open road evaluation.

Faster speed-of-processing seemed to enable adults to react better to unexpected events that require a fast response and to reduce by forty percent the number of dangerous maneuvers on real roads (defined as those that required the training instructor to intervene during the evaluation).

LOOKING AHEAD

Research like this seems to present major opportunities for society. For example, would insurance companies, or the AARP, want to sponsor more research and evaluate whether to offer this type of training to their members? Will major employers see opportunities to improve the performance of older employees by identifying the cognitive skills that may need the most improvement and offering tailored training? We could speculate that a person with faster processing abilities will also be able to make faster decisions and learn faster. Please comment.

That makes sense, based on what we know.

Cognitive abilities evolve in different ways as we age and some typically start to decline in our thirties. Cognitive interventions may help train and improve those abilities and there is already research that strongly indicates where and how training can be useful. More research is still required to deliver more precise and tailored interventions in a variety of environments. I suspect we will see the field grow significantly - and not just for aging-related priorities. Cognitive training may become useful for a variety of health conditions, such as Parkinson's and Alzheimer's patients, for example. More research will help researchers refine assessments and training programs.

Chapter 6:
Ready for the Future?

The goal of this guide is to help you navigate the emerging, dynamic, field of brain fitness. We hope we have achieved our goal! We also realize that we have raised many questions because of the emerging nature of this field. In particular, we cannot "prescribe" specific brain training programs: we can just offer the most relevant and updated information, and leave it up to you, the informed consumer or professional, to exercise your brain and make appropriate decisions.

In this final chapter our aim is to describe the trends we think are important in order to help you be ready for the future. Consumers will be more and more aware that brain health is critical for healthy and successful aging. Informed and proactive adults will look for solutions to integrate brain fitness to their everyday activities. Professionals will identify opportunities to offer new services and programs. We hope this chapter will give you ideas as to how to introduce brain fitness in your personal life and/or your workplace.

6.1. BRAIN FITNESS GOES MAINSTREAM

Increased emphasis on brain maintenance

The emphasis on brain maintenance will increase in locations ranging from retirement communities to gyms. As a computer-savvy adults population looks for ways to stay mentally fit, brain fitness, or brain training, is becoming part of their vocabulary and concern.

However, for this to happen, higher quality research will need to back up specific interventions. The need for independent studies is strong. Indeed, published research of cognitive training interventions has so far been sponsored and/or conducted by the companies themselves. As Dr Arthur Kramer says: "We need … a kind of independent "seal of approval" based on independent clinical trials" (see Dr. Kramer's interview at the end of Chapter 2).

Integration of physical and mental exercise

Today physical and mental exercise usually take place in very different settings: the former, in health clubs, the later, in universities or at home. We predict that the borders between them will become more diffuse.

Expect new programs such as brain fitness podcasts that allow us to train working memory as we jog or exercise bikes with built-in brain games.

Broad government initiatives

Government initiatives to increase public awareness of the need for brain fitness will be launched. It is becoming more widely understood by the medical and public policy communities that a combination of physical exercise, nutrition, mental exercise and stress management can help us maintain our brain health as we age. As politicians and policy makers look for ways to delay the onset of Alzheimer-related symptoms and other dementias in our aging population, new initiatives may be launched.

Initiatives are underway. Dr. Daniel Gopher explains that he is involved in a new research project labeled "Skills-multimodal interfaces for the capturing and transfer of skills" (see Dr. Gopher's interview at the end of Chapter 5). This project aims at facilitating and improving the acquisition and transfer of skills using virtual-reality multimodal interfaces. It is supported by the European Commission: 15 industry and university research partners, from nine countries, are involved.

The government of Ontario, Canada, has invested $10 m to create a Brain Fitness Centre at Baycrest Research Institute to develop brain fitness applications that can be distributed through their healthcare channels.

6.2. LEVERAGING BETTER TOOLS

Assessment of cognitive functions

Better and more widely available assessments of cognitive function will serve as objective baselines to measure the impact of cognitive training interventions. There will also likely be better diagnostic tests to identify early symptoms of dementia. Reliable diagnostic assessments of cognitive abilities will help move this field forward just as jumping on a scale is helpful in telling you if your physical fitness and diet program is working.

It may sound like science-fiction but serious initiatives are underway. Dr. Arthur Kramer explains how The National Institute of Health is preparing an "NIH Toolbox". This toolbox aims at providing reliable instruments that researchers and clinicians could all use, instead of using many different, non-comparable, measures. This initiative was launched in 2006 and is a five years effort.

Computer-based tools to improve clinical conditions

Better computer-based tools to improve clinical conditions will appear. The growing pipeline of research studies will enable the market leaders and new entrants to refine existing tools and devise new ones. More clinical studies will show the benefits of brain fitness programs to address specific clinical conditions and learning disabilities.

Dr. Jerri Edwards points out that although more research is needed to deliver tailored interventions, cognitive training may become increasingly useful for a variety of health conditions, such as Parkinson's disease and Alzheimer's type dementia (see Dr. Edwards' interview at the end of Chapter 5).

Some of the ongoing studies are in the following areas:

- Schizophrenia: Dr. Sophia Vinogradov from the University of California at San Francisco was awarded a $1.1 million grant from National Institute of Mental Health in 2005 (unpublished results as of February 2008). The aim of the study is to investigate the efficacy of computerized cognitive training exercises on the remediation of cognitive deficits associated with schizophrenia. Participants are assigned randomly to receive treatment with either computerized cognitive training or commercially available computer games.

- Alzheimer's Disease: An ongoing NIH study led by Dr. Joel Kramer and Kristine Yaffe of University of California at San Francisco aims at evaluating the effects of a computer-based training program ("HiFi-AD") on the memory and cognitive abilities of individuals diagnosed with mild Alzheimer's Type Dementia.
- Autism: TeachTown is a computer-assisted instruction program that utilizes practices such as ABA to teach a variety of skills to children with autism. Promising preliminary results published in 2006 by Waren and her colleagues showed that the use of the software successfully enhanced social communication and decrease inappropriate behaviors. The same team is currently conducting research funded by the U.S. Department of Education.
- Cancer: Chemotherapy for cancer is associated with a number of negative side effects. One of these side effects is a deficit in cognitive function, a condition commonly referred to as "chemobrain". Cognitive decline is often reported to affect memory, attention, executive functions and processing speed. Posit Science and Lumosity are being used in separate ongoing NIH trials to evaluate whether cognitive training can accelerate the rehabilitation needed to address the cognitive effects of chemotherapy.

Low-tech options

Low tech options will play an increasing role in the brain fitness field. Already, increasing research is showing the cognitive value and brain plasticity impact of interventions such as meditation and cognitive therapy (see Chapter 3). More research and wider applications will help refine our understanding of when and how they can be most helpful.

The future years will see a great increase in the number of older adults. The consequent cognitive declines presented by patients in several medical institutions may overwhelm the healthcare system. It will be important for health practitioners to keep current on the different techniques available to deal with cognitive decline. High-tech, computerized, techniques may not always be the answer. Low-tech, more accessible, solutions may be of great utility to professionals like nurses who interact daily with older adults (see the article by Vance and colleagues published in 2008 in *The Journal of Neuroscience Nursing*)

The school system will play a role in the development of low-tech methods of brain training. As Dr. James Zull explains, "If I had to select one mental muscle that students should really exercise and grow during their school years, I would say they need to build their "learning muscle" – to learn how to learn" (see Dr. Zull's interview in Chapter 1).

6.3. A GROWING ECOSYSTEM

Psychologists and physicians

Psychologists and physicians will have to help patients navigate through the overwhelming range of available products and interpret the results of cognitive assessments. Indeed, according to Dr. Larry McCleary (whose interview you will find at the end of Chapter 2), health professionals should counsel their patients on tips for brain health in the same way they discuss cardiac risk factors and how to address them.

However, as Dr. Arthur Lavin points out, many professionals were educated in the days when scientists still believed that the brain was not much plastic and rather "un-trainable" (see Dr. Lavin's interview at the end of Chapter 3). As a consequence, these professionals are quite skeptical regarding brain fitness and its potential benefits. Significant professional development efforts will be required.

Insurance companies

Insurance companies will introduce incentives for members to encourage healthy aging. Many insurance plans today include rewards for members who, for example, voluntarily take health-related questionnaires that enable them to identify steps to take to improve health. Increasingly, brain-related lifestyle factors will become part of these interventions.

Companies like Allstate have already taken proactive measures to reduce driving risks in older drivers by offering their Pennsylvania members aged 50-75 to participate in a training program involving the Insight software. If this initiative is successful Allstate plans to use the program nationwide and perhaps even offer discounts to policy-holders who commit to using the program.

U.S. military

As the military increasingly funds research to improve the diagnostic and treatment of problems such as Post-Traumatic Stress Disorder and Traumatic Brain Injury, the resulting products will ultimately find commercial uses.

For instance, Dr. Arthur Kramer's lab is involved in a five years study for the U.S. Navy to explore ways to capitalize on emerging research about brain plasticity to enhance training and performance. The MIT and Dr. Kramer's lab will be looking for the best ways to increase the efficiency and efficacy of training of individual and team performance skills. They will focus on skills requiring high levels of flexibility. Dr. Kramer points out that the results from this study will be in the public domain, where they will contribute to the growth of the field of brain fitness in general (see Dr. Kramer's interview in Chapter 2).

Corporate America

Brain fitness will be added to corporate wellness and leadership initiatives. Large employers with existing corporate wellness and leadership programs will introduce brain fitness specific programs aimed not only at improved health outcomes but also at increased productivity and cognitive performance in the workplace.

Dr. Daniel Gopher, whose interview is reported in Chapter 5, describes what process one would follow to develop applications for specific activities or professions: "First, one needs to analyze what cognitive skills are involved in playing at top level, and then develop a computer-based cognitive simulation that trains those skills. What most people do not realize is that top players are not born top players. We are not just talking about instincts. We are talking about skills that can be trained."

6.4. CONCLUSIONS

The main message behind the discovery of brain plasticity is that the way we live our life can affect how well our brain age. This is great news. However there is no just one general solution to brain maintenance. Science suggests so far to take a multi-pronged approach centered around balanced nutrition, stress management, and both physical and mental exercise.

Brain training, defined as the structured use of cognitive exercises or techniques aimed at improving specific brain functions, can be delivered in a number of ways: meditation, cognitive therapy, cognitive training. The field is still emerging and many more controlled and randomized studies are needed to (a) assess individuals' cognitive profiles easily, (b) validate the effects of different brain training programs, (c) compare different types of brain trainings, (d) assess the appropriateness of certain types of brain trainings for certain specific populations.

One crucial aspect of brain training that needs much improvement is the baseline cognitive screening. Tools that allow the user to assess his or her brain functions before the training starts are necessary for sound brain training. They would allow the consumer or patient to target the specific brain functions that do need training.

Does brain training work? It depends how "work" is defined. If it is defined as quantifiable short-term improvements after a number of weeks of systematic brain training to improve specific cognitive skills, then yes. A number of the brain fitness software programs on the market today do seem to work. If, on the other hand, "working" means measurable long-term benefits, such as better overall brain health as we age, or lower incidence of dementia symptoms, then the answer is that circumstantial evidence suggests they may work. But it is still too early to tell definitively.

Brain training is becoming more and more popular and may play an increasing role in our everyday life in future years. It is easy to get lost in the increasing number of products available. This is why staying informed is crucial! Consumers need to learn how to evaluate their cognitive needs and how to find the right product to match their need. Our hope is to be able to help you along the way.

Chapter 7.

Opening the Debate

The goal of this guide is to inform you, but also to stimulate discussion. In this final chapter we want to provide you, the ambassadors of brain fitness and lifelong learning, with additional food for though.

7.1. THE CASE FOR SOCIAL ENGAGEMENT

You may remember the answer of Dr. Art Kramer in Chapter 2 when asked about the top key lifestyle habits that help delay Alzheimer's symptoms and improve overall brain health: "Ideally, combine both physical and mental stimulation along with social interactions. Why not take a good walk with friends to discuss a book?"

This is why you will find below a few questions to help you delve deeper into the topics discussed in *The SharpBrains Guide*. We suggest that you discuss these questions with your friends, loved ones, the members of your book club, at a meeting of fellow professionals, etc.

Thinking about the questions by yourself would be a stimulating intellectual exercise but discussing the questions with a group of people would boost the power of this brain exercise. Indeed, recent findings suggest that social contact may help us improve our brain functions. For instance, in 2008, Ybarra and his colleagues randomly assigned participants (aged 18-21) to three groups: 1) a social group, in which the participants engaged in a discussion of a social issue for 10mn, 2) an intellectual activities group, in which the participants solved stimulating tasks (crossword puzzles and the likes) for 10mn, and 3) a control group, in which the participants watched a 10mn clip of Seinfeld. After they participated in the discussion or watched the clip or solved the puzzles, the cognitive functioning of all the participants was assessed. Two tasks were used (a speed of processing task and a working memory task).

Results of Ybarra's study showed that people in the intellectual activities group did better in the cognitive tasks than people who merely watched a movie. This suggests that stimulating activities are good for your brain. The benefit from social interaction was as great as the benefit from intellectual activities! This is a very exciting result considering that participants engaged in discussion for only 10 minutes.

Why would social interaction boost brain function? Ybarra and colleagues offer the following reasoning. Social interaction involves many behaviors that require memory, attention and control. These mental processes are also involved in many cognitive tasks. Thus social interaction would act as a prime, it would "oil" these processes so that they are ready to be used when a cognitive task is to be solved. This is a tentative explanation that may require some refinement but the results are here: Social interaction seems to benefit the brain.

By writing this guide, we have done our best to contribute to your good brain health and cognitive fitness. Now it is your turn.

7.2. BOOK CLUB DISCUSSION GUIDE

Book: *The SharpBrains Guide to Brain Fitness* by Alvaro Fernandez and Dr. Elkhonon Goldberg

Description: *The SharpBrains Guide* combines expert, independent advice with 18 in-depth interviews with scientists to present a thought-provoking and informative perspective on the importance of brain fitness. This is the first book to offer guidance on how to navigate the growing amount of brain fitness-related research and products.

You can use these book club discussion questions to help your book club, friends or colleagues delve deeper into the topics discussed in *The SharpBrains Guide* and, along the way, contribute to our collective brain fitness.

1. What have you been doing over the last couple of years to help maintain your brain in top shape?
2. Please describe what you have learned about your brain that has surprised you the most.
3. Before reading this book, what did you think about what "Use It or Lose It" mean? And what do you think now?
4. Why do we, as a society, often pay more attention to car maintenance (cleaning, check-ups, gas, oil changes…) than to how to maintain our brains in good shape? Will this change, and why or why not?
5. What are some of the main mental abilities to nurture beyond memory? And why may doing so result in a better memory?
6. What interviews did you enjoy the most? Why do some scientists say things that seem to contradict what other scientists say?
7. Is the brain value of doing 25 crossword puzzles different depending on whether those are our first ever 25 puzzles or whether we already have done 10,000 puzzles before? Why?
8. What are some types of mental exercise or brain training, and what may they be best for?
9. Do you feel better equipped now to understand, compare and evaluate the claims of different products? How could this guide be improved?
10. How can this emerging field of brain fitness affect the way you perform your job in the future?

We invite you to submit your answers to these questions via the Contact Us form in www.SharpBrains.com. At the end of every month we will review all answers submitted and, with your permission, publish the best answers in SharpBrains.com.

Glossary

Brain Fitness: the general state of feeling alert, in control, productive. Having the mental abilities required to function in society, in our occupations, in our communities.

Brain Training or Cognitive training: structured set of brain exercises, either computer-based or not, designed to train specific brain areas and functions in targeted ways.

Chronic Stress: ongoing, long-term stress. Continued physiological arousal where stressors interfere with neural function and negatively impact the immune system's defenses.

Cognitive Abilities (or Brain functions): brain-based skills we need to carry out any task. They have more to do with the mechanisms of how we learn, remember, and pay attention rather than with any actual knowledge. Examples are memory, attention, and language skills.

Cognitive Reserve (or Brain Reserve): theory that addresses the fact that individuals vary considerably in the severity of cognitive aging and clinical dementia. Mental stimulation, education and occupational level are believed to be major active components of building a cognitive reserve that can help resist the effects of brain disease on cognition.

Cognitive therapy: type of therapy based on the idea that the way people perceive their experience influences their behaviors and emotions. The therapist teaches the patient cognitive and behavioral skills to modify his or her dysfunctional thinking and actions. CT aims at improving specific cognitive skills or behaviors (such as planning and mental flexibility), as well as at helping the individual combat the symptoms and undesirable effects of clinical conditions (such as depression, obsessive-compulsive disorders, or phobias).

Executive Functions: Abilities that enable goal-oriented behavior, such as the ability to plan, and execute a goal. These include flexibility, theory of mind, anticipation, self-regulation, working memory and inhibition.

Neurogenesis: the process by which neurons continue to develop all throughout our lives.

Neuroimaging: techniques that either directly or indirectly image the structure, function, or physiology of the brain. Recent techniques (such as fMRI) have enabled researchers to understand better the living human brain.

Neuroplasticity: the brain's ability to reorganize itself throughout life.

PubMed: very useful tool to search for published studies. PubMed is a service of the U.S. National Library of Medicine that includes over 16 million citations from MEDLINE and other life science journals for biomedical articles back to the 1950s. It includes links to full text articles and other related resources.

Working memory: the ability to keep information current for a short period while using this information. Working memory is used for controlling attention, and deficits in working memory capacity lead to attention problems.

References

INTRODUCTION

- Basak, C. et al. (2008). Can training in a real-time strategy video game attenuate cognitive decline in older adults? *Psychology and Aging.*
- Begley, S. (2007). *Train your mind, change your brain: How a new science reveals our extraordinary potential to transform ourselves.* Ballantine Books.
- DeKosky, S. T., et al. (2008). *Ginkgo biloba* for prevention of dementia: a randomized controlled trial. *Journal of the American Medical Association, 300,* 2253-2262.
- Doidge, N. (2007). *The Brain that changes itself: Stories of personal triumph from the frontiers of brain science.* Viking Adult.

CHAPTER 1

- Bunge, S. A., & Wright, S. B. (2007). Neurodevelopmental changes in working memory and cognitive control. *Current Opinion In Neurobiology, 17*(2), 243-50.
- Damasio, A. (1995). *Descartes' error: Emotion, reason, and the human brain.* Penguin Press.
- David Kolb, D. (1983). *Experiential learning: Experience as the source of learning and development.* FT Press.
- Draganski, B., Gaser, C., Kempermann, G., Kuhn, H. G., Winkler, J., Buchel, C., & May A. (2006). Temporal and spatial dynamics of brain structure changes during extensive learning. *The Journal of Neuroscience, 261231,* 6314-6317.
- Gage, F. H., Kempermann, G., & Song, H. (2007). *Adult Neurogenesis.* Cold Spring Harbor Laboratory Press, NY.
- Gardner, H. (1983). *Frames of Mind: The theory of multiple intelligences.* New York: Basic Books.

- Gaser, C. & Schlaug, G. (2003). Brain structures differ between musicians and non-musicians. *The Journal of Neuroscience, 23*, 9240-9245.

- Jensen, E. (2006). *Enriching the brain: How to maximize every learner's potential.* Jossey-Bass.

- Klingberg, T., Fernell, E., Olesen, P. J., Johnson, M., Gustafsson, P., Dahlström, K., Gillberg, C. G., Forssberg, H., & Westerberg, H. (2005). Computerized Training of Working Memory in Children With ADHD-A Randomized, Controlled Trial. *J American Academy of Child and Adolescent Psychiatry, 44*(2), 177-186.

- Maguire, E. A., Woollett, K., & Spiers, H. J. (2006). London taxi drivers and bus drivers: A structural MRI and neuropsychological analysis. *Hippocampus, 16*, 1091-1101.

- Mechelli, A., Crinion, J. T., Noppeney, U. , O'Doherty, J., Ashburner, J., Frackowiak, R. S., & Price, C. J. (2004). Structural plasticity in the bilingual brain. *Nature, 431*, 757.

- Parsons, L. M. (2001). Exploring the functional neuroanatomy of music performance, perception, and comprehension. *Annals Of The New York Academy Of Sciences, 930*, 211-31.

- Roenker, D., Cissell, G., Ball, K., Wadley, V., & Edwards, J. (2003). Speed of processing and driving simulator training result in improved driving performance. *Human Factors, 45*, 218-233.

- Rueda, M. R., Posner, M. I., & Rothbart, M. K. (2005) The development of executive attention: contributions to the emergence of self-regulation. *Developmental Neuropsychology, 28*, 573-594.

- Rueda, M. R., Rothbart, M. K.., Saccamanno, L., & Posner, M. I. (2005) Training,maturation and genetic influences on the development of executive attention. *Proceedings of the National Academy of Sciences, 102,* 14931-14936.

- Stern, Y. (2002). What is cognitive reserve? Theory and research application of the reserve concept. *Journal of Int. Neuropsych. Soc., 8*, 448-460.

- Sylwester, R. (2007). *The adolescent brain: Reaching for autonomy.* Corwin Press.

- Tang, Y., Ma, Y., Wang, J., Fan, Y., Feng, S., Lu, Q., et al. (2007). Short-term meditation training improves attention and self-regulation. *Proceedings of the National Academy of Sciences, 104*(43), 17152-17156.
- Woodruff, L., & Woodruff, B. (2007). *In an instant: A Family's journey of love and healing.* Random House.
- Zull, J. E. (2002). *The art of changing the brain: Enriching the practice of teaching by exploring the biology of learning.* Stylus Publishing.

CHAPTER 2

- Ball, K., Berch, D. B., Helmers, K. F., Jobe, J. B., Leveck, M. D., Marsiske, M., Morris, J. N., Rebok, G. W., Smith, D. M., Tennstedt, S. L., Unverzagt, F. W., & Willis, S. L. (2002). Effects of cognitive training interventions with older adults. *Journal of the American Medical Association, 288,* 2271-2281.
- Basak, C. et al. (2008). Can training in a real-time strategy video game attenuate cognitive decline in older adults? *Psychology and Aging.*
- Brooks, J. O., Friedman, L., Pearman, A. M., Gray, C., & Yesavage, J. A. (1999). Mnemonic training in older adults: Effect of age, length of training, and type of cognitive pretraining. *International Psychogeriatrics, 11,* 75-84.
- Burns, N. R., Bryan J., Nettelbeck T. (2006). Ginkgo biloba: no robust effect on cognitive abilities or mood in healthy young or older adults. *Human Psychopharmacology, 21*(1), 27-37.
- Colcombe, S., & Kramer, A. F. (2003). Fitness effects on the cognitive function of older adults: A Meta-Analytic study. *Psychological Science,* 14 (2) , 125–130.
- DeKosky, S. T., et al. (2008). *Ginkgo biloba* for prevention of dementia: a randomized controlled trial. *Journal of the American Medical Association, 300,* 2253-2262.
- Derwinger, A., Neely, A. S., Persson, M., Hill, R. D., & Backman, L. (2003). Remembering numbers in old age: Mnemonic training versus self-generated strategy training. *Aging Neuropsychology and Cognition, 10,* 202-214.

- Elsabagh, S., Hartley, D. E., Ali, O., Williamson, E. M., & File, S. E. (2005). Differential cognitive effects of Ginkgo biloba after acute and chronic treatment in healthy young volunteers. *Psychopharmacology, 179*(2), 437-46

- Eriksson, P. S., Perfilieva, E., Bjork-Eriksson, T., Alborn, A. N., Norborg, C., Peterson, D., & Gage, F. H. (1998). Neurogenesis in the adult human hippocampus. *Nature Medicine, 4*(11): 1313-1317, 1998.

- Faherty, C. J., Shepherd, K. R., Herasimtschuk, A., & Smeyne, R. J. (2005). Environmental enrichment in adulthood eliminates neuronal death in experimental Parkinsonism. *Molecular Brain Research, 134*(1), 170-179.

- Fontani, G., Corradeschi, F., Felici, A., Alfatti, F., Migliorini, S., & Lodi L. (2005). Cognitive and physiological effects of Omega-3 polyunsaturated fatty acid supplementation in healthy subjects. *European Journal of Clin. Invest., 35*(11), 691-9.

- Gage, F. H., Kempermann, G., & Song, H. (2007). *Adult Neurogenesis.* Cold Spring Harbor Laboratory Press, NY.

- Gopher, D., Weil, M., & Bareket, T. (1994). Transfer of skill from a computer game trainer to flight. *Human Factors, 36*, 1-19.

- Heyn, P., Abreu, B. C., & Ottenbacher, K. J. (2004). The effects of exercise training on elderly persons with cognitive impairment and dementia: a meta-analysis. *Archives of Physical Medicine and Rehabilitation, 85*(10), 1694-704.

- Hillman, C. H., Erickson, K. I., & Kramer, A. F. (2008). Be smart, exercise your heart: exercise effects on brain and cognition. *Nature Reviews Neuroscience 9* (1), 58-65.

- Katzman, R., Aronson, M., Fuld, P., Kawas, C., Brown, T., Morgenstern, H., Frishman, W., Gidez, L., Eder, H., & Ooi, W.L. (1989). Development of dementing illnesses in an 80-year-old volunteer cohort. *Annals of Neurology, 25*, 317–324.

- McCleary, L. (2007).*The Brain Trust Program: A scientifically based three-part plan to improve memory, elevate mood, enhance attention, alleviate migraine and menopausal symptoms, and boost mental energy.* Perigee Trade.

- McCraty, R., Barrios-Choplin, B., Rozman, D., Atkinson, M., & Watkins, A. D. (1998). The impact of a new emotional self-management program on stress, emotions, heart rate variability, DHEA and cortisol. *Integr. Physiol. Behav. Sci., 33*(2), 151-70.
- Nair, K. S., Rizza, R. A., O'Brien, P., Dhatariya, K., Short, K. R., Nehra, A., Vittone, J. L., et al. (2006). DHEA in elderly women and DHEA or testosterone in elderly men. *The New England Journal of Medicine, 355*(16), 1647-59.
- Piscitelli, S. C, Burstein, A. H., Chaitt, D., Alfaro, R. M., Falloon, J. (2001). Indinavir concentrations and St John's wort. *Lancet, 357,* 1210.
- Roenker, D., Cissell, G., Ball, K., Wadley, V., & Edwards, J. (2003). Speed of processing and driving simulator training result in improved driving performance. *Human Factors, 45,* 218-233.
- Sapolsky, R. M. (2004). *Why zebras don't get ulcers.* Owl Books.
- Scarmeas, N., Levy, G., Tang, M. X., Manly, J., & Stern, Y. (2001). Influence of leisure activity on the incidence of Alzheimer's disease. *Neurology, 57,* 2236-2242.
- Snowdon, D. A., Ostwald, S. K., Kane, R. L., & Keenan, N. L. (1989). Years of life with good and poor mental and physical function in the elderly. *Journal of Clinical Epidemiology, 42,* 1055-1066.
- Solomon, P. R, Adams, F., Silver, A., Zimmer, J., & DeVeaux, R. (2002). Ginkgo for memory enhancement: a randomized controlled trial. *JAMA, 288*(7), 835-40.
- Stern, Y. (2002). What is cognitive reserve? Theory and research application of the reserve concept. *Journal of Int. Neuropsych. Soc., 8,* 448-460.
- Verhaeghen, P., Marcoen, A., & Goosens, L. (1992). Improving memory performance in the aged through mnemonic training: A meta-analytic study. *Psychology and Aging, 7,* 242-251.
- Willis, S. L., Tennstedt, S. L., Marsiske, M., Ball, K., Elias, J., Koepke, K. M., Morris, J. N., Rebok, G. W. Unverzagt, F. W. Stoddard, A. M., & Wright, E. (2006). Long-term effects of cognitive training on everyday functional outcomes in older adults. *Journal of the American Medical Association, 296*(23), 2805-2814.

- Wilson, R.S., Bennett, D.A., Bienias, J.L., Aggarwal, N.T., Mendes de Leon, C.F., Morris, M.C., Schneider, J. A., & Evans, D. A. (2002). Cognitive activity and incident AD in a population-based sample of older persons. *Neurology, 59*, 1910-1914.
- Zelinski et al. (on-going). The IMPACT Study: A randomized controlled trial of a brain plasticity-based training program for age-related decline.
- Zelinski, E. M., & Burnight, K. P. (1997). Sixteen-year longitudinal and time lag changes in memory and cognition in older adults. *Psychology and Aging, 12*(3), 503-513.
- Zull, J. E. (2002). *The Art of changing the brain: Enriching the practice of teaching by exploring the biology of learning.* Stylus Publishing: Sterling, VA.

CHAPTER 3

- American Society on Aging (2006). ASA-Metlife Foundation Attitudes and Awareness of Brain Health Poll.
- Basak, C. et al. (2008). Can training in a real-time strategy video game attenuate cognitive decline in older adults? *Psychology and Aging.*
- Beck, A. (1979). *Cognitive therapy and the emotional disorders.* Plume.
- Beck, J. S. (1995). *Cognitive Therapy: Basics and Beyond.* Guilford Press.
- Beck, J. S. (2007). *The Beck diet solution: Train your brain to think like a thin person.* Oxmoor House.
- Ericsson, K. A., & Delaney, P. F. (1998). Working Memory and Expert Performance. In R. H. Logie & K. J. Gilhooly (Eds.), *Working Memory and Thinking*, pp. 93-114. Hillsdale, NJ: Erlbaum.
- Gaab, N, Gabrieli, J. D. E., Deutsch, G. K., & Temple, E. (2007). Neural correlates of rapid auditory processing are disrupted in children with developmental dyslexia and ameliorated with training: An fMRI study. *Restorative Neurology and Neuroscience, 25*, 295-310.
- Gopher, D., Weil, M., & Baraket, T. (1994). Transfer of skill from a computer game trainer to flight. *Human Factors, 36*, 387-405.

- Hambrick, D. Z., Sathouse, T. A., & Meinz, E. J. (1999). Predictors of crossword puzzle proficiency and moderators of age-cognition relations. *Journal of Experimental Psychology: General, 128*, 131-164.

- Hillman, C. H., Erickson, K. I., & Kramer, A. F. (2008). Be smart, exercise your heart: exercise effects on brain and cognition. *Nature Reviews Neuroscience* 9 (1), 58-65.

- Jaeggi, S. M., Buschkuehl, M., Jonides, J., & Perrig, W. J. (2008). Improving fluid intelligence with training on working memory. *Proceedings of the National Academy of Sciences of the United States of America, 105*(19), 6829-6833.

- Jobe, J. B., Smith, D. M., Ball, K., Tennstedt, S. L., Marsiske, M., Willis, S. L., Rebok, G. W., Morris, J. N., Helmers, K. F., Leveck, M. D., Kleinman, K. (2001). ACTIVE: A cognitive intervention trail to promote independence in older adults. *Control Clinical Trials, 22*(4), 453-479.

- Kawashima, R. (2005). *Train your brain: 60 days to a better brain.* Kumon Publishing North America.

- Klingberg, T., Fernell, E., Olesen, P. J., Johnson, M., Gustafsson, P., Dahlström, K., Gillberg, C. G., Forssberg, H., & Westerberg, H. (2005). Computerized training of working memory in children with ADHD- A randomized, controlled trial. *J. American Academy of Child and Adolescent Psychiatry, 44*(2), 177-186.

- Lavin, A., & Glaser, S. (2006). *Who's boss: Moving families from conflict to collaboration.* Collaboration Press.

- Lavin, A., & Glaser, S. *(2007). Baby and toddler sleep solutions for dummies.* Wiley.

- Levine, M. (1995). *All kinds of minds.* Educators Publishing Service

- Mahncke, H. W., Connor, B. B., Appelman, J., Ahsanuddin, O. N., Hardy, J. L., Wood, R. A., Joyce, N. M., Boniske, T., Atkins, S. M., & Merzenich, M. M. (2006). Memory enhancement in healthy older adults using a brain plasticity-based training program: A randomized, controlled study. *PNAS, 103*(33), 12523-12528.

- Davidson, R. J., Kabat-Zinn, J., Schumacher, J., Rosenkranz, M., Muller, D., Santorelli, S. F., Urbanowski, F., Harrington, A., Bonus, K.

and Sheridan, J. F. (2003). Alterations in brain and immune function produced by mindfulness meditation. *Psychosomatic Medicine, 65,* 564-570.

- Newberg, A., D'Aquili, E., & Rause, V. (2001). *Why God won't go away: Brain science and the biology of belief.* Ballantine Books.

- Newberg, A. & Waldman, M. R. (2006). *Why we believe what we believe: Uncovering our biological need for meaning, spirituality, and truth.* Free Press.

- Paquette, V., Levesque, J., Mensour, B., Leroux, J. M., Beaudoin, G., Bourgouin, P., et al. (2003). Effects of cognitive-behavioral therapy on the neural correlates of spider phobia. *Neuroimage, 18,* 401-409.

- Roenker, D., Cissell, G., Ball, K., Wadley, V., & Edwards, J. (2003). Speed of processing and driving simulator training result in improved driving performance. *Human Factors, 45:* 218-233.

- Scarmeas, N., Levy, G., Tang, M. X., Manly, J., & Stern, Y. (2001). Influence of leisure activity on the incidence of Alzheimer's disease. *Neurology, 57,* 2236-2242.

- Stahre, L., Tärnell, B., Håkanson, C.-.E., & Hällström, T. (2007). A randomized controlled trial of two weight-reducing short-term group treatment programs for obesity with an 18-month follow-up. *International Journal of Behavioral Medicine, 14*(1), 48-55

- Steenbarger, B, N. (2006). *Enhancing Trader Performance: Proven Strategies From the Cutting Edge of Trading Psychology.* Wiley.

- Steenbarger, B. N. (2003). *The Psychology of Trading: Tools and Techniques for Minding the Markets.* Wiley.

- Tang, Y., Ma, Y., Wang, J., Fan, Y., Feng, S., Lu, Q., et al. (2007). Short-term meditation training improves attention and self-regulation. *Proceedings of the National Academy of Sciences, 104*(43), 17152-17156.

- Temple, E., Deutsch, G. K., Poldrack, R. A., Miller, S. L., Tallal, P.,Merzenich, M. M., & Gabrieli, J. D. E. (2003). Neural deficits in children with dyslexia ameliorated by behavioral remediation: Evidence from functional MRI. *Proc. Natl. Acad. Sci. USA, 100,* 2860-2865.

- Willis, S. L., Tennstedt, S. L., Marsiske, M., Ball, K., Elias, J., Koepke, K. M., Morris, J. N., Rebok, G. W. Unverzagt, F. W. Stoddard, A. M., &

Wright, E. (2006). Long-term effects of cognitive training on everyday functional outcomes in older adults. *Journal of the American Medical Association, 296*(23), 2805-2814.

- Woodruff, L., & Woodruff, B. (2007). *In an Instant: A Family's journey of love and healing.* Random House.
- Zelinski et al. (on-going). The IMPACT Study: A randomized controlled trial of a brain plasticity-based training program for age-related decline.

CHAPTER 4

- Baril, L., Nicolas, L., Croisile, B., Crozier, P., Hessler, C., Sassolas, A., McCormick, J. B., & Trannoy, E. (2004). Immune response to Abeta-peptides in peripheral blood from patients with Alzheimer's disease and control subjects. *Neurosci. Lett., 355*(3), 226-30
- Gopher, D., Weil, M., & Bareket, T. (1994). Transfer of skill from a computer game trainer to flight. *Human Factors, 36*, 1-19.
- Kawashima, R. (2005). *Train your brain: 60 days to a better brain.* Kumon Publishing North America.
- Klingberg, T., Fernell, E., Olesen, P. J., Johnson, M., Gustafsson, P., Dahlström, K., Gillberg, C. G., Forssberg, H., & Westerberg, H. (2005). Computerized training of working memory in children with ADHD-A randomized, controlled trial. *J. American Academy of Child and Adolescent Psychiatry, 44*(2), 177-186.
- Mahncke, H. W., Connor, B. B., Appelman, J., Ahsanuddin, O. N., Hardy, J. L., Wood, R. A., Joyce, N. M., Boniske, T., Atkins, S. M., & Merzenich, M. M. (2006). Memory enhancement in healthy older adults using a brain plasticity-based training program: A randomized, controlled study. *PNAS, 103*(33), 12523-12528.
- Nussbaum, P. (2007). *Your brain health lifestyle.* Word Association.
- Small, G. (2005). *The memory prescription: Dr. Gary Small's 14-day plan to keep your brain and body young.* Hyperion.
- Steenbarger, B, N. (2006). *Enhancing trader performance: Proven strategies from the cutting edge of trading psychology.* Wiley.

CHAPTER 5

- Barkley, R. A. (1997). Attention-deficit/hyperactivity disorder, self-regulation, and time: Toward a more comprehensive theory. *Journal of Developmental & Behavioral Pediatrics, 18*(4), 271-279.
- Centers for Disease Control and Prevention and the Alzheimer's Association. (2007). *The Healthy Brain Initiative: A National Public Health Road Map to Maintaining Cognitive Health.*
- Cicerone, K. D., Dahlberg, C., Kalmar, K., Langenbahn, D. M., Malec, J. F., Bergquist, T. F., Felicetti, T., Giacino, J. T., Harley, J. P., Harrington, D. E., Herzog, J., Kneipp, S., Laatsch, L., & Morse P. A. (2000). Evidence-based cognitive rehabilitation: recommendations for clinical practice. *Arch. Phys. Med. Rehabil., 81*, 1596-615.
- Cicerone, K. D., Dahlberg, C., Malec, J. F., Langenbahn, D. M., Felicetti, T., Kneipp, S., Ellmo, W., Kalmar, K., Giacino, J. T., Harley, J. P., Laatsch, L., Morse, P. A., & Catanese, J. (2005). Evidence-based cognitive rehabilitation: Updated review of the literature from 1998 through 2002. *Arch. Phys. Med. Rehabil., 86*, 1681-92.
- Goldstein, S., & Ingersoll, B. (1993). Controversial treatments for children with ADHD and impulse disorders. In L. F., Koziol C. E. Stout, and D. Ruben, (Eds.). *Handbook of childhood impulse disorders and ADHD: Theory and practice.* Charles C Thomas, Publisher, pp. 144-160
- Gopher, D., Weil, M., & Baraket, T. (1994). Transfer of skill from a computer game trainer to flight. *Human Factors, 36*, 387-405.
- Kasten, E., Wuest, S., Behrens-Bamann, W., & Sabel, B. A. (1998). Computer-based training for the treatment of partial blindness. *Nature Medicine, 4*, 1083–1087.
- Klingberg, T., Fernell, E., Olesen, P. J., Johnson, M., Gustafsson, P., Dahlström, K., Gillberg, C. G., Forssberg, H., & Westerberg, H. (2005). Computerized training of working memory in children with ADHD-A randomized, controlled trial. *J. American Academy of Child and Adolescent Psychiatry, 44*(2), 177-186.
- Mark Katz, M. (1997). *On playing a poor hand well.* W.W. Norton and Company.

- Olesen, P. J., Westerberg, H., & Klingberg, T. (2004). Increased prefrontal and parietal brain activity after training of working memory. *Nature Neuroscience, 7*(1), 75-79.
- Rabiner, D., & Coie, J. D. (2000). Early attention problems and children's reading achievement: A longitudinal investigation. *Journal of the American Academy of Child & Adolescent Psychiatry, 39*(7), 859-867.
- Roenker, D., Cissell, G., Ball, K., Wadley, V., & Edwards, J. (2003). Speed of processing and driving simulator training result in improved driving performance. *Human Factors, 45*, 218-233.
- Shebilske, W. L., Volz, R. A., Gildea, K. M., Workman, J. W., Nanjanath, M., Cao, S,, & Whetzel, J. (2005). Revised Space Fortress: A validation study. *Behavior Research Methods, 37*, 591-601.
- Willis, S. L., Tennstedt, S. L., Marsiske, M., Ball, K., Elias, J., Koepke, K. M., Morris, J. N., Rebok, G. W. Unverzagt, F. W. Stoddard, A. M., & Wright, E. (2006). Long-term effects of cognitive training on everyday functional outcomes in older adults. *Journal of the American Medical Association, 296*(23), 2805-2814.

CHAPTER 6

- Whalen, C., Liden, L., Ingersoll, B., Dallaire, E., & Liden, S. (2006). Positive behavioral changes associated with the use of computer-assisted instruction for young children. *Journal of Speech and Language Pathology and Applied Behavior Analysis, 1*(1), 11-25.
- Vance, D. E., Webb, N. M., Marceaux, J. C., Viamonte, S. M., Foote, A. W., & Ball, K. K. (2008). Mental stimulation, neural plasticity, and aging: directions for nursing research and practice. *Journal of Neuroscience Nursing, 40*(4), 241-9.

CHAPTER 7

- Ybarra, O., Burnstein, E., Winkielman, P., Keller, M. C., Manis, M., Chan, E., & Rodriguez, J. (2008). Mental exercising through simple socializing: Social interaction promotes general cognitive functioning. *Personality and Social Psychology Bulletin, 34*, 248-259.

About SharpBrains

SharpBrains is the leading market research and advisory services firm covering the growing number of education and healthcare applications of cognitive science and neuroscience. SharpBrains' mission is to provide individuals, companies and institutions with independent, high-quality, research-based, information and guidance to navigate the growing cognitive and brain fitness market. The firm publishes an annual series of market reports, titled the State of the Brain Fitness Software Market, for executives and investors.

Alvaro Fernandez is co-founder and CEO of SharpBrains. He received masters' in education and business from Stanford University, and teaches at UC-Berkeley Osher Lifelong Learning Institute. A member of the World Economic Forum's Global Agenda Councils, he has been quoted in *The New York Times*, CNN, and more.

Dr. Elkhonon Goldberg is renowned for his clinical work, research, and teaching. Co-founder and Chief Scientific Advisor of SharpBrains, he is also a Clinical Professor of neurology at New York University School of Medicine and the author of *The Executive Brain: Frontal Lobes and The Civilized Mind* and *The Wisdom Paradox: How Your Mind Can Grow Stronger as Your Brain Grows Older.*

SharpBrains.com (http://www.sharpbrains.com/), the firm's educational blog and website, offers many helpful and free resources, including:

- Hundreds of searchable articles
- A free monthly newsletter
- A blog with frequent new articles written by SharpBrains staff and over 15 expert contributors
- Brain teasers
- Checklists and other tools
- Recommended books
- Recommended websites

All the available resources are frequently updated to make sure that you stay current. We hope you visit us!

Index